The functional psychoses continue to be classed as illnesses of unknown origin, and the validity of diagnostic concepts therefore depends on extrinsic criteria such as course and outcome, results of biological and genetic investigation, and response to treatment. 'Operational' diagnostic criteria are the main subject of this book, which presents a comprehensive review of the present state of diagnostic formulations for functional psychoses.

From the early nosological and pathogenetic concepts of Kraepelin, Bleuler, Schneider and Kasanin, the authors trace the development, internationally, of the various classifications of the functional psychoses, culminating among others in those embodied in the latest ICD and DSM formulations.

This is a revised and expanded edition of 'Diagnostic Criteria for Schizophrenic and Affective Psychoses' and is also published under the auspices of the World Psychiatric Association. Diagnostic criteria have been selected for inclusion on the basis of their historical importance, their influence on current diagnostic systems, their international scope and their scientific importance. The authors provide an indispensible commentary on the 'Babel of differing formulations in psychiatric diagnosis', and urge a new 'polydiagnostic' approach to psychiatric research, in a book that will be of the greatest value to clinicians and scientific investigators alike.

T0243045

Diagnostic criteria for functional psychoses

Diagnostic criteria
for
functional psychoses

P. Berner
E. Gabriel
H. Katschnig
W. Kieffer
K. Koehler
G. Lenz
D. Nutzinger
H. Schanda
C. Simhandl

SECOND EDITION

Published under the auspices of the
World Psychiatric Association

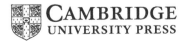
CAMBRIDGE
UNIVERSITY PRESS

CAMBRIDGE UNIVERSITY PRESS
Cambridge, New York, Melbourne, Madrid, Cape Town, Singapore, São Paulo

Cambridge University Press
The Edinburgh Building, Cambridge CB2 2RU, UK

Published in the United States of America by Cambridge University Press, New York

www.cambridge.org
Information on this title: www.cambridge.org/9780521423151

First published by the World Psychiatric Association 1983, as
Diagnostic criteria for schizophrenic and affective psychoses
Second edition published by Cambridge University Press 1992

This digitally printed first paperback version 2006

A catalogue record for this publication is available from the British Library

Library of Congress Cataloguing in Publication data

Diagnostic criteria for functional psychoses / P. Berner . . .
[et al.]. – 2nd ed.
  p.   cm.
Rev. ed. of: *Diagnostic criteria for schizophrenic and affective psychoses* /
P. Berner . . . [et al.]. c 1983
Includes bibliographical references.
ISBN 0–521–42315–5 (hardback)
1. Psychoses – Diagnosis.   2. Schizophrenia – Diagnosis.
3. Manic depressive psychoses – Diagnosis.
4. Schizoaffective disorders – Diagnosis.
5. Paranoia – Diagnosis.   I. Berner, P. (Peter)
II. Diagnostic criteria for schizophrenic and affective psychoses.
[DNLM: 1. Psychotic Disorders – classification.
2. Psychotic Disorders – diagnosis.   WM 202 D536]
RC512.D475   1992
616.89′075 – dc20   91–29347   CIP

ISBN-13 978-0-521-42315-1 hardback
ISBN-10 0-521-42315-5 hardback

ISBN-13 978-0-521-03512-5 paperback
ISBN-10 0-521-03512-0 paperback

CONTENTS

Contents

Contents

Contents

AUTHORS

P. Berner, MD

Professor of Psychiatry
Formerly head, Psychiatric Clinic
University of Vienna
1090 Vienna, Währinger Gürtel 18–20, Austria

E. Gabriel, MD

Professor of Psychiatry
Head, Psychiatric Hospital of Vienna
1140 Vienna, Baumgartner Höhe 1, Austria

H. Katschnig, MD

Professor of Psychiatry
Head, Psychiatric Clinic
University of Vienna
1090 Vienna, Währinger Gürtel 18–20, Austria

W. Kieffer, MD

Assistant Professor of Psychiatry
Psychiatric Clinic
University of Vienna
1090 Vienna, Währinger Gürtel 18–20, Austria

K. Koehler, MD

Professor of Psychiatry
Psychiatric Clinic
University of Bonn
53000 Bonn 1, Sigmund Freud Strasse 25, Germany

G. Lenz, MD

Associate Professor of Psychiatry
Psychiatric Clinic
University of Vienna
1090 Vienna, Währinger Gürtel 18–20, Austria

D. Nutzinger, MD

Associate Professor of Psychiatry
Psychiatric Clinic
University of Vienna
1090 Vienna, Währinger Gürtel 18–20, Austria

H. Schanda, MD   Associate Professor of Psychiatry
                      Medical Director of Justizanstalt
                      Göllersdorf
                      2013 Göllersdorf, Schlossgasse 17, Austria

C. Simhandl, MD   Assistant Professor of Psychiatry
                      Psychiatric Clinic
                      University of Vienna
                      1090 Vienna, Währinger Gürtel 18–20, Austria

PREFACE

During the past fifteen years, the use of operational criteria for diagnosis in psychiatry assumed an ever increasing importance. The World Psychiatric Association felt consequently called upon to prepare an easily accessible review of diagnostic formulations and made the results of this work available for the occasion of the VII World Congress of Psychiatry held in 1983. The scope of the book published at that time in English and German, and subsequently followed up by Spanish (1986), Japanese (1986), and French (1987) editions was, however, restricted to schizophrenia and major affective disorders.

The success of the English version of those 'Diagnostic criteria for schizophrenic and affective psychoses' (Berner *et al.*, 1983a) called for an effort to extend the content of the second edition to cover the entire group of 'Functional Psychoses'. A greater number of authors was therefore employed on compilation of the second edition whose title reflects the added material. Whereas the first edition reviewed and evaluated a number of diagnostic criteria systems for schizophrenic and affective psychoses only, this new publication includes criteria pertaining also to schizoaffective and paranoid psychoses. We selected the criteria on the basis of their historical importance, their effect on currently applied diagnostic systems, their use in many parts of the world, and their scientific foundation. We crave the reader's understanding for the fact that, owing to limited space, we were obliged to concentrate on the systems prominently in use. Our commentaries, however, cover also a number of the lesser known ones. Some of the criteria systems already contained in the first edition have, since 1983, been further developed and supplemented, and these modifications have been taken into account in compilation of the second edition. The diagnostic and statistical manual of mental disorders (DSM-III) criteria, for instance, has been supplemented by the DSM-III-R formulations; the April 1989 provisional draft for the international classification of diseases (ICD-10) which, in due time, will supercede the ICD-9 is also referred to in our material; and the French empirical diagnostic criteria, of which only provisional definitions for non-affective disorders were available at the time of the first edition in 1983, are now presented in their definitive form. An operational definition 'for non-specific depressive syndrome' is also provided.

We had to remember that terminology may vary according to school and language. Consequently, in this book 'functional' and 'endogenous' are used synonymously, as are in like manner 'affective' or 'manic-depressive' psychoses and 'cyclothymia', as well as 'paranoid' and 'delusional' psychoses. The book's contents are arranged in the following way:

1. An introduction (part A) presents on the one hand a historical review of the diagnostic principles concerning functional psychoses and, on the other, the foundations for a new research strategy, the 'polydiagnostic approach'.
2. The four principal sections of the book follow: after a few preliminary comments, 17 diagnostic criteria systems for schizophrenic (Chapters B1-17), 13 for affective (Chapters C1-13), 7 for schizoaffective (Chapter D1-7), and 10 for paranoid psychoses (Chapters E1-10).
3. The description of each diagnostic system begins with a presentation of its criteria in tabular form, either quoted from the original publication* or assembled or translated by us.† Where Criteria sections are quoted the appropriate source is given as a footnote. The ensuing commentary consists of a brief account of the system's background; the criteria composing it are then described and analyzed on the basis of their logical structure.
4. The chapters on affective, schizoaffective, and paranoid psychoses (parts C, D, and E) do not always repeat relevant information already discussed in part B (schizophrenic psychoses). Instead, the reader is referred to these earlier discussions.
5. Citations can be found in part F, the bibliography, at the end of the book.

This book is not intended as an ersatz for the original literature. Rather, by comparing the various diagnostic formulations, we hope to promote interest for the problems of classification so important to research and clinical practice. We also hope to stimulate interest in the original literature and encourage greater understanding among the various psychiatric schools.

We thank the readers and users of the 'Diagnostic criteria for schizophrenic and affective psychoses' for their suggestions for improvement which have been taken into account in this second edition, whose readers and users we encourage to proceed in the same way.

---

* In the quoted material, 'he' is sometimes used in the general sense.

† For ease of cross-reference, attempts have been made to preserve the layout and style of the Criteria sections.

A

INTRODUCTION

The functional psychoses continue to be classed as illnesses of unknown origin. Diagnostic concepts for this category can be considered only as hypotheses, the validity of which depends on extrinsic criteria such as course and outcome, genetic data, response to treatment, and results of biological investigation. The requirement for validation is that the procedure for diagnostic attribution in question be set up in an unequivocal and reproducible manner. The operational diagnostic criteria, which have been developed primarily within the last fifteen years, issue from this concern.

Our intentions in presenting this collection of diagnostic criteria are twofold: first, to offer a comprehensive view of the present state of diagnostic formulations for functional psychoses; second, to encourage greater involvement in a 'polydiagnostic approach' (Berner and Katschnig, 1983) to psychiatric research, an endeavor consisting of the simultaneous application of as many diagnostic criteria as possible to the same patient population. After rendering a brief historical account of the principles which have governed diagnosis in our area of concern, this introductory chapter goes on to present the polydiagnostic approach.

Functional psychoses, principles of diagnosis

Kraepelin, building on the knowledge of his French and German predecessors and taking course and outcome of morbid states as the most important guidelines, presented the fundamentals of his psychiatric nosology in 1899. He conceived dementia praecox and manic-depressive illness as the main categories of disorders of unknown origin, but maintained paranoia – and in some elaborations of his classification also paraphrenia – as separate entities. This concept established the frame in which all further divergent developments with regard to the differential diagnosis of functional psychoses took place, a process fueled by the search for criteria permitting a cross-sectional diagnosis instead of relying

1

on a long-term observation. These developments were centered around two basic problems that are still reflected in the various classificatory approaches presented in this book. The first one concerns the diagnostic distinction between dementia praecox, for which Bleuler's term 'schizophrenia' soon became the habitual denomination, and manic-depressive illness. It requires not only a clear decision as to which symptomatological or other criteria should be regarded as characteristic for schizophrenic and affective disorders but also raises the question of whether cases presenting a simultaneous or consecutive combination of schizophrenic and manic-depressive features should be attributed to the former or latter category or be regarded as an independent 'schizoaffective' disorder. The second problem relates to the maintenance of functional psychoses as entities distinct from the schizophrenic, manic-depressive, or – if this diagnosis is accepted – schizoaffective category. The most important subject of disagreement in this respect has always been the nosological independence of certain delusional disorders. The different standpoints with regard to this question and the etio-pathogenetic considerations sustaining them are discussed in the sections on paranoid and schizoaffective psychoses.

A historical review of the attempts to propose solutions for the differential diagnostic problems outlined above demonstrates that their basic requirement is a clear concept as to how schizophrenia and manic-depressive illness should be defined. Although Kraepelin, because of the emphasis he put on course and outcome, came up with no obligatory symptoms for his categories, his description of dementia praecox and manic-depressive insanity already contained most of the criteria which were to serve later as a matrix for the selection of cross-sectional symptoms determining diagnosis. For the most part, subsequent contributions to the description of these illnesses have served only to complete and to define more precisely their symptomatology. In this respect the precise definition of schizophrenia appeared to be the most delicate problem; subsequently, classic psychiatric literature had concerned itself far more with the definition of this disorder than with diagnostic problems linked to affective psychoses.

Eugen Bleuler's (1911) distinction between basic and accessory symptoms represents a first step in the direction of operational criteria in this field, whereby basic symptoms are drawn upon for cross-sectional diagnosis of schizophrenia. Bleuler also replaced Kraepelin's nosological hypothesis with a pathogenetic one. This states that various etiologies – finally taken by Bleuler as well as Kraepelin to be of somatic nature – may lead to those pathogenetic stages which manifest through characteristic basic symptoms. These basic symptoms, however, are not considered to be the immediate expression of the supposed underlying somatic process but essentially to represent 'mechanisms' through which the patient tries to cope with the disturbances of brain function. 'Primary symptoms' emanating directly from the somatic process are thus, in Bleuler's opinion, difficult to perceive in the clinical picture. He therefore recommends that diagnosis be established by means of basic symptoms. The suspicion that some of them may be completely nonspecific subsequently instigated several schools to select for diagnostic purposes only those basic symptoms which seemed to reflect at least to a certain degree the underlying 'primary disturbances,' among which Bleuler assigns special importance to the 'dissociation' of psychic functions. In this perspective formal thought disorders or inappropriate affect acquired a specific diagnostic weight in some systems. These symptoms are frequently used to demarcate schizophrenic from non-schizophrenic delusional disorders.

Drawing upon Kraepelin's concept of dementia praecox as a deteriorating process, many authors also refer to affective blunting for the same purpose in spite of the fact that this feature – although belonging to the basic symptoms – is considered by Bleuler to be a purely secondary mechanism.

Kurt Schneider (1939) established a pragmatic system for assessing schizophrenic symptoms. His point of departure is based on Karl Jaspers' (1963) distinction between disturbances of experience and disturbances of behavior. Since the former are much easier to grasp, Schneider built his diagnostic system mainly on them, separating these disturbances of experience into two categories: first rank symptoms and second rank symptoms. Schizophrenic disturbances of thought, affect, and contact with others are behavioral; therefore Bleuler's basic symptoms were divested of nearly all their diagnostic and theoretical weight, for Schneider maintained that his rules for diagnostic classification were based exclusively on psychopathological evaluation. From this position one often deduces that Schneider's diagnostic procedure is atheoretical, purely pragmatic. This conclusion is only partly true: Kurt Schneider never gave reason to doubt that he supported the endogeny theory (Moebius, 1893), which, although avoiding any etiological or pathogenetic commitments, does consider functional psychoses to be constitutionally predetermined in the long run.

Another theoretical element in the Schneiderian system concerns the differentiation between cyclothymia* (denomination by which Schneider replaces the term 'manic-depressive illness') and schizophrenia, whereby Jaspers' (1913, 1946) hierarchical principle (of 'levels') comes into play. This principle is based on the assumption that neurotic symptoms or personality disorders are relatively 'superficial,' whereas affective, schizophrenic, and organic symptoms lie deeper. When several symptoms

* Throughout this book cyclothymia is used as a synonym for endogenous affective disorder.

which belong to various 'levels' occur simultaneously or consecutively, diagnosis is determined by the deepest 'level' reached. The hierarchical principle is accepted by many schools as a guideline for distinguishing functional psychoses from neurotic, personality, or organic disorders. Opinion is currently very divided, however, over the hierarchical relationship between affective and schizophrenic symptoms, and this situation is reflected by differences in modern diagnostic criteria.

The application of the hierarchical principle to differentiate between schizophrenia and manic-depressive illness leaves, of course, no room for schizoaffective disorders. Therefore, when forwarding his concept of 'schizoaffective psychoses' in America, Kasanin (1933) had to abolish Jaspers' (1963) principle, a standpoint which is maintained as a distinct category in all systems comprising these disorders.

The observation that the illness of patients diagnosed as schizophrenic according to Bleuler's criteria did not always follow an unfavorable course led Langfeldt (1937, 1939, 1956) to search for criteria which could distinguish between a bona fide 'process schizophrenia' and 'schizophreniform psychoses' having a good prognosis. Many Scandinavian authors, finding that the latter often manifested as a result of triggering life events, felt that these 'schizophreniform psychoses' should at least in part be considered 'psychogenic' disorders. The concept of 'psychogenic psychoses' introduced in Scandinavia by Wimmer (1916) linked well with the reflections of German authors such as Gaupp (1910) and Kretschmer (1950), who suggested that some delusional disorders could, at least partially, be of psychogenic origin. These considerations do not at all deny the possibility of the existence of independent non-schizophrenic and non-manic-depressive endogenous psychoses. But Kasanin's and Langfeldt's publications stimulated considerably the search for a more precise definition of schizophrenia.

Whatever the nosological position of the schizoaffective psychoses may be, Kasanin found that such cases frequently followed a benign course. This prompted supporters of the Kraepelinian dementia praecox concept to draw upon the affective components of these patients' symptomatology and any additionally ascertainable non-symptomatological particularities as well for the discrimination from genuine nuclear schizophrenia. The contributions of Kasanin and Langfeldt instigated the elaboration of partly symptomatological and partly non-symptomatological indicators for a favorable and unfavorable prognosis. The former have become incorporated into many operational systems for diagnosis of schizophrenia as *exclusion criteria*, the latter as *inclusion criteria*.

Recent investigations, such as those reported by Pope and Lipinski (1978), Koehler (1979), Pope *et al.* (1980), and Berner (1982), prompted a number of researchers to assume that schizophrenic, and not affective, symptoms had no differential diagnostic weight for distinguishing between schizophrenia and cyclothymia. This idea is tantamount to a reversal of the hierarchical principle; the consequence of its application is that not only current but also previous cyclothymic symptoms and perhaps even a positive family history for major affective disorder will be used as excluding criteria for the diagnosis of schizophrenia. This leads, though, to the notion that schizophrenic symptoms in general are fully non-specific phenomena which may appear under various 'psychotic conditions.' Diagnostic procedures taking this point of view into account will give schizophrenic symptoms a positive rating solely when not only organic and affective but also psychogenic disorders can be excluded.

A theoretical explanation for the non-specificity of at least part of the 'classic' schizophrenic symptoms has been provided by Janzarik (1959) in his concept of the 'structural-dynamic coherency model'. Since this appears to be an important and fertile approach for finding solutions to the problem of differentiating between schizophrenic and affective psychoses, it will be mentioned here in greater detail. Janzarik designated as 'dynamic' a fundamental realm embracing affectivity and drive, which he contrasted with the 'psychic structure' containing behavior patterns and representations (cognitive notions), both inborn and acquired largely throughout the developmental period. Parts of this structure become dynamically invested, meaning that they are connected with positive, negative, or ambivalent feelings. Those markedly invested or 'dynamically loaded' parts of the structure are called 'values' and comprise the 'value structure'.

'Dynamics' however, are not entirely tied to structural elements. Everybody has at his disposal a certain amount of 'free floating dynamics,' subject to alterations called basic dynamic constellations. When attaining a level of morbidity, these modifications correspond either to 'dynamic depletion,' seen clinically as affective blunting, or to 'dynamic derailments.' There are three types of derailment: dynamic 'expansion', as in mania, 'restriction', as in depression, and 'instability', characterized by rapid fluctuations or 'swings' between the first two states. Dynamic derailments affect an actualization of specific values: in states of expansion, for example, the positive elements of the structure are actualized, while in states of restriction the negative ones prevail, since positive values find no actualization. In states of dynamic instability, rapid changes in actualization of differently invested parts of the structure occur, whereby 'ambivalently' invested elements of the value structure also become conscious. Higher levels of instability lead to 'delusional impressions'*, delusional perceptions, illusions, and hallucinations. The

---

* 'Delusional impressions' (*Anmutungserlebnisse*) resemble delusional mood in that one's surroundings are felt to be changed in a way that is striking and puzzling. In the former, however, these changes are limited to certain perceived objects or details thereof.

rapid swings in drive, emotional resonance, and affectivity are over-powering, making one feel at their mercy; this may explain how feelings of will-deprivation, alien influence, depersonalization, derealization, and ambivalence arise.

In the light of this theory, dynamic instability appears to be the source of Schneider's first rank symptoms and a part of Bleuler's basic symptoms. Janzarik's assumption that the dynamic instability may arise in abnormal mental conditions, stemming from various origins, creates doubts as to the specificity of these phenomena. These suspicions were also strength-ened by a series of investigations (those reported by Mellor (1982), for example). In particular, experiences with rapidly alternating, 'unstable' manic-depressive mixed states (Carlson and Goodwin, 1973; Nunn, 1979), which the school of Hamburg calls *'Mischbilder'* (or 'mixed pictures', Mentzos, 1967), and with *'bouffées délirantes'* (Magnan, 1893) support the point of view that instability, giving rise to the aforementioned symptoms, occurs often in affective psychoses.

In contrast to schizophrenia, whose definition since Kraepelin had continually been the subject of scientific disagreements and new attempts at formulation, the original concepts of mania and melancholia by Falret (1854), Baillarger (1854), and Kraepelin (1913) were generally accepted without a murmur. Only since the development of operational criteria for attribution to psychiatric diagnoses during the last decade have the affective psychoses again become a subject of discussion, centering on three main points: the delimitation from schizophrenia, the distinction between unipolar and bipolar affective psychoses, and the differentiation between subtypes in depression.

Kasanin (1933) and Janzarik (1959) can be regarded as forerunners of the current discussion on the discrimination of affective disorders from schizo-phrenia. Leonhard (1957), Angst (1966), and Perris (1966) have made important contributions to the bipolar–unipolar dichotomy hypothesis.

In the middle of the 1960s two groups of authors developed scales for distinguishing between an endogenous (psychotic) type and a reactive (neurotic) type of depression on the basis of the two-type hypothesis (Newcastle scale (NCS), Carney *et al.*, 1965; depressive category type scale (DCTS), Sandifer *et al.*, 1966). The endogenous/non-endogenous dicho-tomy led to a second Newcastle scale (Gurney, 1971). Since the first Newcastle scale serves as a basis for the French diagnostic criteria for depression and both of them are widely used, they are included along with the French criteria among this book's criteria.

Also worthy of mention is that, on the basis of empirical evidence and theoretical considerations (Jung, 1952), biorhythmic disturbances are taken into several definitions. The distinction between primary and secondary disturbances introduced in the early 1970s (Robins *et al.*, 1972) is to be considered as a purely pragmatic principle of attribution.

If one tries to group the particular elements of the various diagnostic criteria for endogenous psychoses with respect to the reasons leading to their selection, one can schematically distinguish between theory-oriented pragmatic and empirical approaches. The most important theoretical concepts are:

1. The endogeny hypothesis
2. Kraepelin's nosological hypothesis based on course and outcome
3. Bleuler's pathogenetic primary disturbance hypothesis for schizophrenia
4. Jaspers' hierarchical principle
5. Janzarik's model of structural-dynamic coherency
6. The biorhythmic disturbance hypothesis for affective psychoses
7. The bipolar–unipolar dichotomy hypothesis

Examples for pragmatic approaches are Kurt Schneider's (1939) hierarchy of disturbances of experience and Robins' distinction between primary and secondary affective disorders (Robins *et al.*, 1972). Empirical elements are, above all, those criteria which have proved their worth on the basis of past validation studies (for example, prognostic indicators). Conditions under which criteria normally taken as relevant cannot be given a positive rating (such as blunting of affect when very tired) also belong here.

All criteria for diagnosis presented in this book contain elements stemming from various approaches. Depending on which elements are employed and in which combination the diagnostic instrument in question puts them together, the patient population selected will vary. Consequently, the commentaries on the particular systems will refer to the fundamental considerations and hypotheses mentioned in this introduction.

The polydiagnostic approach in psychiatric research

The simultaneous use of several diagnostic formulations embracing one and the same patient population in psychiatric research projects was dubbed the 'polydiagnostic approach' by Berner and Katschnig (1983). This approach was systematically developed at the Psychiatric Clinic of the University of Vienna and pursued in several research projects during the late seventies and early eighties (Berner *et al.*, 1983*c*; Katschnig, 1984*a*; Katschnig, 1984*b*; Katschnig and Berner, 1985). During the same period many publications applying the same principle have appeared in England and in the USA (Brockington *et al.*, 1978; Overall and Hollister, 1979; Helzer *et al.*, 1981; Stephens *et al.*, 1982; Young *et al.*, 1982; Endicott *et al.*, 1982; Kendell, 1982). In the last few years the 'polydiagnostic approach' has been further elaborated by us (Katschnig and Seelig, 1985; Katschnig *et al.*, 1986*a*, *b*; Berner *et al.*, 1986*b*, *c*; Lenz *et al.*, 1986; Katschnig and Simhandl, 1986).

The polydiagnostic approach represents, in our point of view, a new paradigm in psychiatric research, which can contribute to the solution of many controversies and to the resolution of many contradictions in the results of research to date.

The 'Babel of differing formulations in psychiatric diagnosis' (Brockington *et al.*, 1978) prompted the elaboration of compromise classification systems – achieved only after a great deal of effort – at national and international levels. It was hoped that these compromises would enable a standardization of psychiatric diagnostics in even larger regions or throughout the world. The prototype of these compromise classification systems is the international classification of diseases of the World Health Organization (WHO), whose 9th revision appeared in 1978 (ICD–9, 1978) and whose 10th revision is under way (ICD–10, 1989*a*, *b*). The American Psychiatric Association developed its own compromise classification system parallel to the ICD–9, the diagnostic and statistical manual of mental disorders, now in its third revised edition (DSM–III–R, 1987). Both these classification systems suffer from all the imperfections inherent in any compromise: for reasons of general and psychiatric policy, conflicting positions and formulations had to be incorporated into each system often at the expense of clarity, theory and logic. That 'operational definitions' for phenomena leading to diagnosis appear here and there, and inclusion and exclusion criteria are defined, should not be misleading in this respect (Berner *et al.*, 1983*b*).

The compromise character of these large diagnostic systems makes them unsuitable for psychiatric research. However, diagnostic formulations developed by just a few authors or small research groups are as a rule much more logically construed, although they may at the same time be biased by their ideology. Nevertheless, when one considers such formulations as hypotheses accessible to scientific evaluation, the one-sidedness of their contents becomes less important. It has also proved possible to examine the same patient population employing various diagnostic formulations for a given illness concept, for example for schizophrenia, and thus to investigate the various correlations existing between 'factors' and various definitions of the same concept. That is what we mean by the 'polydiagnostic approach.'

Katschnig *et al.* (1986*b*) were able to show that the relationship between life events and subtypes of depression depended primarily on the particular diagnostic formulation of the subtypes of depression. Not only life events but also other 'factors' such as the dexamethasone suppression test, genetic factors, or illness course could be investigated concerning their relationship to various definitions of the same illness concept (Davidson *et al.*, 1984*a*; Schanda *et al.*, 1986; Katschnig *et al.*, 1986*a*). Such a procedure enables comparison with other investigations which have used only one specific diagnostic system for patient selection. Moreover, for generalizing the validity of the results of research projects, comparable results obtained by means of the application of various diagnostic formulations serve as confirmatory evidence; conflicting results using different diagnostic formulations call for a more reserved appreciation.

Another suitable application of the polydiagnostic approach concerns the analysis of the contents and logic of specific diagnostic formulations. The approach could become a kind of 'comparative psychiatric nosology' fostering a greater mutual understanding among psychiatrists in different countries and cultures. Thus it should be possible to diminish gradually, on a worldwide scale, the differences in psychiatric diagnostics.

The polydiagnostic approach may look rather cumbersome at first glance, for it is more difficult to gather a sufficient number of cases if several diagnostic formulations are used simultaneously. Nevertheless, its application has proved to be quite feasible. At the Vienna University Psychiatric Clinic in the late seventies a 'core instrument,' based on the present state examination by Wing *et al.* (1974), was developed for enabling the collection of the basic information needed for all the diagnostic systems to be employed. With the help of this information, a given patient could be diagnosed according to the most diverse diagnostic systems. A computer program had also been developed for the polydiagnostic subclassification of depression into 'endogenous (psychotic)' and 'reactive (neurotic)' types (Katschnig *et al.*, 1981). Recently a more elaborate instrument, called 'polydiagnostic system 2 (PS2)' has been developed which covers all current diagnostic formulations for depression, mania, schizophrenia, schizoaffective disorders, paranoid disorders and anxiety disorders (Katschnig *et al.*, 1987). Results to date have shown that, when the basic requirements of a comprehensive data-gathering 'core instrument' and a computer program have been satisfied, the polydiagnostic approach works.

The application of a single, in many areas also operationally inadequate, compromise diagnostic system may be sufficient for clinical practice and health statistics; for psychiatric research, however, the use of compromise systems should be rejected, because their very nature tends to conceal conflicting views. Therefore, we feel that the simultaneous employment of diagnostic formulations which partly overlap and partly contradict each other is indispensable for the probity and fertility of psychiatric research. The intention of this book is to encourage research workers around the world both to think and to work in a 'polydiagnostic' way and thus to contribute to the growth of a coherent body of knowledge in psychiatry.

B

SCHIZOPHRENIC PSYCHOSES

This section comprises seventeen diagnostic systems. Eleven of them (B6 to B16) can be qualified as operational criteria; the rest really consist only of directives for classification. The first four of the latter were chosen from the abundance of contributions to diagnosis for schizophrenia – not only because they are still widely used but also because, as mentioned in the Introduction, they represent important stages on the path leading to the development of operational criteria. The depiction of these most important foundations for operational criteria is followed by a discussion of the ICD criteria, which represent an international consensus; the criteria of ICD–10 (with respect to the April 1989 draft for the 10th revision) have been operationalized for research purposes.

After the ICD–10 draft come descriptions of all the other operational criteria, arranged according to their degree of relationship. The St Louis criteria (also called the Feighner criteria throughout this book) and the research diagnostic criteria (RDC) are described first of all, followed by the schizophrenia criteria of the DSM–III, which are derived from the Feighner and RDC system, and its successor, the DSM–III–R. Next comes the New Haven schizophrenia index (NHSI), which represents an operational variation of the DSM–III classification scheme. This is succeeded by two systems based on the present state examination (PSE) method; namely the Carpenter–Strauss–Bartko (CSB) system and the CATEGO criteria. The Vienna criteria, which also make use of the PSE for data-gathering, and the Taylor/Abrams criteria, both of which show close ties in their inception, are treated next. The group of operational criteria is completed with the French empirical diagnostic criteria for schizophrenia (Pull *et al.*, 1987*a,b*), which works out the independent path taken by French diagnostic procedure. The classification methods used in the Soviet Union correspond to a course typology; with their discussion this section of the book is brought to a close.

Valid for all systems is that symptoms attributable to an organic illness or to the influence of toxic substances or drugs should not be included as criteria for the functional psychosis in question. Consequently, these symptoms are mentioned explicitly only when figuring as integral elements for exclusion in operational research criteria.

B1

Emil Kraepelin

CRITERIA

I. Symptomatological criteria

- Disturbances of attention and comprehension
- Hallucinations, especially auditory (voices)
- *Gedankenlautwerden* (audible thoughts)
- Experiences of influenced thought
- Disturbances in the flow of thought, above all a loosening of associations
- Impairment of cognitive function and judgment
- Affective flattening
- Appearance of morbid behavior:
  Reduced drive
  Automatic obedience
  Echolalia, echopraxia
  Acting out
  Catatonic frenzy
  Stereotypy
  Negativism
  Autism
  Disturbance of verbal expression

II. Illness course criterion

- Leading to psychic invalidity

COMMENTARY

The disturbances generally accepted at present as syndromatological types of schizophrenic illnesses were described towards the end of the nineteenth century; however, they had not yet been attributed to a particular entity permitting a disengagement from other illnesses. This was accomplished largely through the efforts of Emil Kraepelin. One can follow the evolution of his work in the various editions of his textbook *Psychiatry* starting with the 5th edition, appearing in 1896, and especially from the 6th (1899) to the 8th (1909–1915) editions. His goal was to delineate illnesses having a common cause, symptomatology, course, and outcome. Basing his work on Kahlbaum's (1874) description of catatonia and Hecker's (1871) description of hebephrenia (from which the particular form dementia simplex was later established) and dementia paranoides, he applied the term **dementia praecox** to those illnesses often sharing a similar outcome. This term, first appearing in the 6th edition, was taken from the identical one introduced to French psychiatry by Morel (1860); this school had employed the expression in a purely descriptive sense (see Scharfetter, 1975).

The criteria for Kraepelin's dementia praecox were both symptomatological and evolutional. They were not only to assist in classifying endogenous illnesses but especially to permit a distinction between dementia praecox and manic depressive illness. In the 8th edition published in 1913, the term **paraphrenia** appeared along with dementia praecox in the group of 'endogenous dementias' (*endogene Verblödungen*). This edition was the last one which Kraepelin wrote himself. The following is based on it (and already contains the thought of Eugen Bleuler from 1911).

In 1911 Eugen Bleuler, alluding to the description of dementia praecox and to Kraepelin's accomplishments in general, affirmed: 'He also deserves nearly all the credit for the identification of the various symptoms and their classification' (ibid., p. vii). Three basic features pertaining to different symptom areas distinguish the illness. Morbid states which:

1. 'arise due to inner causes as if out of the blue' (ibid., p. 667), that is, are endogenous
2. 'in the great majority of cases manifest a course leading to a psychic invalidity of varying severity' (ibid., p. 667)
3. 'share an outcome arising from a peculiar destruction of the psychic personality's inner integrity, whereby emotion and volition in particular are impaired' (ibid., p. 668)*
4. On the basis of these changes evidence a great variety of clinical

* Quotations translated from the original German by the authors of this book.

14

pictures occurring in the same patient during the course of his illness,
thus pointing to a common origin

are grouped as dementia praecox. From the observations in his chapter on
endogenous dementias and from his introduction to their principal form,
dementia praecox, one can see that Kraepelin developed the notion of
dementia praecox not only from symptomatology but also from longitudinal and etiological evidence. Out of the description of symptoms he
succeeded in distilling the distinguishing features of a basic disorder and
its various expressions. In the detailed description of symptomatology he
employs the term 'basic disorder' not *sensu stricto* but in a broader sense of
'frequent characteristic symptoms'. Meanwhile, he does not bother
himself with systematic classification into basic and accessory or primary
and secondary symptoms. But, when interpreting particular symptoms,
he does indeed refer to Bleuler's reflections on symptom structure (1911).
The distinction between disturbances of experience and behavior,
respectively reported and observed symptoms of morbidity, however, is
implied in his descriptions – above all in the description concerning the
appearance of morbid behavior; this is preceded by the description of a
number of symptom groups interpretable for the most part as disturbances of experience. It is interesting that his text includes many examples
of performance test results characterizing the disturbance, yet he does not
make diagnostic criteria out of them.

On the basis of what Kraepelin emphasized, one can establish a list of
particularly characteristic symptoms which are presented here as symptomatological diagnostic criteria. Kraepelin's description leads him to the
conclusion that a basic disturbance lies behind the medley of symptoms: it
concerns an 'impoverishment of those feelings and strivings which
continually stoke the furnace of our will,' and a 'loss of the internal
integrity of comprehension, emotion, and volition.' Both these components are intimately related (ibid., p. 746).

A typology of 'disease courses' (clinical subgroups) and outcome
complete this description of the concept of dementia praecox. No other
aspects capable of adding anything to the concept can be found in his
observations because it was Kraepelin's purpose to unite these clinical
forms under the definition. But designating forms of illness whose
affiliation to dementia praecox seemed questionable to him complement
his concept, both psychopathologically and longitudinally speaking,
because they could be separate disease entities similar only in part to
dementia praecox. These disorders are paranoid psychosis, catatonia, late
catatonia, forms manifesting periodicity, and schizophasia (compare with
Chapter C1, Kraepelin's criteria for major affective disorders).

Kraepelin's dementia praecox concept is multiaxial, because three axes
for its determination can be gleaned from the evidence: symptomatological,

longitudinal/course-typological (chronic, leading to psychic invalidity), and etiological (endogenous). Kraepelin himself deemed the term to be provisional because of the limited state of knowledge. A systematic classification of symptoms was not undertaken. Course criterion is of particular import.

Kraepelin's teaching on dementia praecox took on an importance which continues to grow. He grouped the entities formerly described as independent (hebephrenia, catatonia, dementia paranoides, dementia simplex) together as dementia praecox and described their symptoms. These formerly independent entities thus became subgroups (see Chapters B5 and B6, ICD). At the same time he laid the foundation for the further progress of knowledge, for Eugen Bleuler's symptomatological analysis and its growth, and for later attempts to develop multiaxial concepts. The important chapters of the 8th edition of *Psychiatry* were translated promptly into English – the chapters on dementia praecox and paraphrenia already by 1919. Landmark (1982) has taken the initiative to modify Kraepelin's teachings for operational purposes.

B2

Eugen and Manfred Bleuler

I. Symptomatological criteria

Basic or fundamental disturbances

- Formal thought disorders*
- Disturbances of affect*
- Disturbances of the subjective experience of self
- Disturbances of volition and behavior
- Ambivalence*
- Autism*

Accessory symptoms

- Disorders of perception (hallucinations)
- Delusions
- Certain memory disturbances
- Modification of personality
- Changes in speech and writing
- Somatic symptoms
- Catatonic symptoms
- Acute syndromes (such as melancholic, manic, catatonic, and other states)

II. Intensity criterion

- Psychotic (M. Bleuler)

* 'The four A's': association, affect, ambivalence, and autism.

17

COMMENTARY

In 1911 Bleuler introduced the notion of the 'group of schizophrenias' in the title and contents of a volume of Aschaffenburg's *Handbook of Psychiatry*, dedicated to dementia praecox (written in 1908). Referring to Kraepelin (specifically to his *Textbook of Psychiatry*, 7th edition, 1904), Bleuler declared that 'the entire idea of dementia praecox comes from Kraepelin. He also deserves nearly all the credit for the identification and classification of the various symptoms' (ibid., p. VII).* Bleuler stated that the goal of his own contribution is to clarify 'psychological connections' (ibid., p. VII), alluding by this principally to the application of Freud's ideas.

In a very comprehensive first section (ibid., pp. 9–186) describing the symptomatology, he established a distinction between **basic** and **accessory symptoms**. This distinction continues to be applied by the Zürich school (see the editions of the *Textbook of Psychiatry* by Eugen Bleuler, revised by Manfred Bleuler for the past 40 years. The 15th and latest edition appeared in 1983). Demonstration of basic symptoms should lead to the description of those 'specific impairments of thought, affect and relation to one's environment occurring in no-other condition' (Bleuler, 1911, p. 6). Basic symptoms, in contrast to accessory symptoms, are considered to be not only characteristic of the illness but also more or less *permanent* alterations. Only fundamental psychic functions are permanently impaired, not isolated symptoms, and these impairments become all the more pronounced as the illness progresses to an advanced stage. 'Advanced' refers thus to the *degree of impairment* as well. The term 'psychosis,' that is 'insanity,' is taken to define a certain degree of severity (Bleuler, 1983, p. 407). The criterion of the disorder's permanence has been relegated to the background as a result of Manfred Bleuler's longitudinal studies in 1972. Inasmuch as the impairments are not the result of an organic disorder, characteristic schizophrenic symptoms outweigh other psychopathological symptoms, affective ones as well, in terms of nosological importance. However, Manfred Bleuler (1981) concedes a certain position of independence to schizoaffective illnesses within the group of schizophrenias. The hierarchical relation between symptoms arising from an organic disorder and those having no such origin is the result of Eugen Bleuler's having provided for the exclusion of those symptoms 'which play an important role in certain other illnesses, for example (the absence of) primary disturbances of perception, orientation, memory, etc.' as a criterion in the list of basic symptoms (1911, p. 10).

The theoretical, etio-pathogenetic distinction between **primary symptoms,**

* Quotations translated from the original German by the authors of this book.

which are directly related to the illness process and are thus autochthonous, and **secondary symptoms**, which represent reactions to the illness
process and are thus psychologically understandable, is not to be con-
fused with the clinical distinction between basic and accessory symptoms
appearing in schizophrenic illnesses (Bleuler, 1911, pp. 284–370). 'The
primary symptoms are obligatory partial manifestations of an illness. The
secondary ones either may not appear or may undergo modifications
without bearing any influence on the underlying process' (*ibid.*, p. 284).
'Nearly the entire symptomatology of dementia praecox described until
now is a secondary one, ...' (ibid., p. 284) Bleuler suspected primary
symptoms to be:

- Disturbances of association (a weakening or obliteration of thought
  cohesion)
- States of clouded consciousness
- Attacks of mania or melancholia
- Tendency to hallucinate
- Tendency to produce stereotypes
- Various somatic symptoms

In the list of secondary symptoms one finds:

- The brunt of thought disorder
- The disturbance of affect
- Disturbances of memory and orientation
- Automatisms
- Cognitive disturbances
- Depersonalization
- Autism
- Disturbances of volition

It is easy to recognize that the various basic or fundamental symptoms
are not mutually independent: 'all of the separately described expressions
of schizophrenia are intimately related; they are in fact to be understood as
manifestations of a basic personality disturbance' (Bleuler, 1983, p. 409).
Thus it is stated that Bleuler's basic symptoms are derived from a
fundamental disturbance whose existence is hypothesized; however, they
do not represent it. They find expression in disturbances of experience
and behavior. They are revealed in part through the statements of the
patient and in part through the observation of behavior. Other symptomatology is not considered for diagnostic criteria; however, Eugen Bleuler
does make use of the chronological dimension in reference to the stability
of the basic symptoms, and Manfred Bleuler goes further than his father in
emphasizing the importance of intensity: the disorder corresponds to
schizophrenia only if its symptoms reach psychotic magnitude. This does
not suffice for systematic multiaxial purposes. Both father and son do

consider illness probability as a function of the number of characteristic symptoms appearing; however, they do not offer any formalized criteria establishing the number required for its confirmation. (In 1982 Landmark undertook this task for both of them separately).

The paired categories of basic–accessory and primary–secondary symptoms overlap. Whereas Manfred Bleuler has remained true to his father's concept of basic or fundamental symptoms, he has developed a different theory of schizophrenia in which he essentially keeps the distinction between primary and secondary symptoms, yet interprets the illness far more on psychological than on neuropathological grounds.

Application of Bleulerian criteria for the diagnosis of schizophrenia will cross-sectionally cover a broad spectrum of clinical states which coincides to a great extent with the spectrum disclosed by other methods (Bleuler *et al.*, 1976). The Bleulerian concept has significantly influenced international diagnostic habits. This began precociously in 1924 when the first English translation of the *Textbook* (Bleuler, 1983) appeared (the *Handbook* (Bleuler, 1911) was not translated until 1950). Operational criteria have not been formulated; indeed, such criteria would be difficult to conceive of because one is dealing mainly with disorders of function rather than with isolated disturbances. For typical forms of the latter, the concept can serve as a basis for establishing operational criteria. Its elements are to be found in the international classification of diseases (ICD), the St Louis criteria, NHSI, the flexible system for the diagnosis of schizophrenia, the Vienna research criteria, the research diagnostic criteria (RDC), Taylor's criteria, DSM–III, and the French empirical diagnostic criteria for schizophrenia.

B3

Kurt Schneider: first rank symptoms

First rank symptoms

- Audible thoughts
- Voices arguing and/or discussing
- Voices commenting
- Somatic passivity experiences
- Thought withdrawal and other experiences of influenced thought*
- Thought broadcasting
- Delusional perceptions
- All other experiences involving made volition, made affect, and made impulses

Second rank symptoms

- Other disorders of perception
- Sudden delusional ideas
- Perplexity
- Depressive and euphoric mood changes
- Feelings of emotional impoverishment
- And several others as well

* The symptom 'thought insertion' was originally included under other experiences of influenced thought.

COMMENTARY

Ever since 1939, Kurt Schneider has promoted his teachings of mental status and psychiatric diagnosis. This represents the essence of his book

Clinical Psychopathology, which first appeared in 1950. One finds therein that he has summarized his own contributions to psychiatry very concisely. The book's teaching is based on the psychopathological concepts of the Heidelberg school at that time; these were summarized in the famous volume on schizophrenia of the *Bumke Handbook*, edited by Wilmanns (1932).

Schneider presented those 'disturbances of experience appearing in schizophrenia' as *'first rank symptoms*, not because we took them for "basic disturbances" but because they possess considerable weight as criteria for diagnosis, not only non-psychotic forms of mental abnormality but also cyclothymia'* (1959, p. 135†). Schneider then emphasizes that the symptoms were chosen exclusively because of their diagnostic, especially their differential typological, weight, thus contrasting his own with Bleuler's (1983) basic–accessory and primary–secondary symptoms. Schneider's is a **pragmatic** approach, thus including only those symptoms 'whose conceptual comprehension and clinical recognition present no undue difficulty' (ibid., p. 136). They are, without exception, disturbances of experience reported by the patient. Some of these symptoms concern modes of experience mutually stemming from a disturbance in an underlying structure corresponding to ego-functioning (thought withdrawal, other experiences of influenced thought, thought broadcasting, and everything having to do with feelings, impulses, and intentions which the patient feels are being 'made'). Accession to first rank status, however, is not determined in reference to an underlying structure or similar etiological and/or pathogenetic considerations. Schneider did not regard first rank symptoms as obligatory requirements for the diagnosis of a schizophrenic illness. Such a decision may also find support from the presence of second rank symptoms and disturbances of expression.

In any case, only symptoms corresponding to psychopathological status are taken as diagnostic criteria; other indications such as syndromes, illness course, and personality traits are not enlisted. Etiopathogenetic support plays only a minor role, inasmuch as the existence of organicity is considered to exclude the diagnosis of schizophrenia. First rank symptoms are taught to be a pragmatic instrument for the differential typology of endogenous psychoses; 'when confronted with the undisputable presence of such disturbances of experience, we make in all modesty the clinical diagnosis of schizophrenia provided no organicity can be found' (ibid., p. 135); however, they are not intended as a theoretical instrument. This pragmatic approach is thus qualified because the first rank symptoms themselves are not universally applicable; that is, they

---

* 'Cyclothymia' is used here and elsewhere as a synonym for major affective disorder.

† These and subsequent quotations translated by the authors of this book from the latest (12th) edition, unrevised since the 8th edition.

possess differential typological value only in the absence of organic psychosis. If such be the case, first rank symptoms *prevail* over all others – affective symptoms as well. In case first rank symptoms have made their appearance *at any time* during the course of an illness, the diagnosis of schizophrenia will be established and maintained.

Schneider knows of cases for which the differential typological distinction between schizophrenia and cyclothymia fails and calls them 'cases in-between' (ibid., p. 114). Using second rank as well as first rank criteria in such cases, he can speak of more or less atypical cases of schizophrenia – only in connection with cyclothymia, naturally. The boundary separating schizophrenia from non-psychotic mental abnormality, however, is sharply drawn in as much as first rank symptoms are taken to be endogenous.

Application of first rank symptoms for the diagnosis of schizophrenia will cross-sectionally cover a broad spectrum of clinical states which coincides to a great extent with the spectrum disclosed by other criteria (Bleuler *et al.*, 1976). The teaching of diagnosing schizophrenic illnesses with the help of first rank symptoms has exerted a great deal of influence worldwide thanks to translations in almost all the principal languages of the world (first English edition in 1959, before that, see Schneider 1950; first French edition in 1957; first Spanish edition in 1951, among others) and numerous German re-editions. The international pilot study of schizophrenia (IPSS; WHO, 1973) has revealed, by means of statistical group comparisons, that first rank symptoms do discriminate between schizophrenia and cyclothymia on an international level; however, they are apparently not employed in the way Schneider had intended, namely in accordance with the hierarchical principle, as prevailing differential typological evidence in each case of non-organic psychosis (Carpenter and Strauss, 1974; Carpenter *et al.*, 1973*b*). First rank symptoms play an important role in many subsequent elaborations of diagnostic criteria, such as in the international classification of diseases (ICD), the CSB system, RDC, the Taylor/Abrams criteria, and in the diagnostic and statistical manual, third edition (DSM–III) of the American Psychiatric Association.

First rank symptoms were the first implements for an operational definition of schizophrenia. The relative ease with which they can be comprehended and identified was one of the motives behind Schneider's choice. They possess a high clinical relevance, which is why they have taken on considerable influence in German- and English-speaking countries. Their shortcomings lie in their heterogeneity and their lack of reliance on a hypothesized basic disturbance. The majority of them appear in Bleuler's accessory symptoms.

B4

Gabriel Langfeldt

I. Symptomatological criteria

Significant clues to a diagnosis of schizophrenia are (if no sign of organic brain disorder, infection or intoxication can be demonstrated):

(a) Changes in personality, which manifest themselves as a special type of emotional blunting followed by lack of initiative, and altered, frequently peculiar behavior. (In hebephrenia especially these changes are quite characteristic and are a principal clue to the diagnosis)

(b) In catatonic types the history as well as the typical signs in periods of restlessness and stupor (with negativism, oily facies, catalepsy, special vegetative symptoms, etc.)

(c) In paranoid psychoses essential symptoms of split personality (or 'depersonalization symptoms') and a loss of reality feeling ('derealization symptoms') or primary delusions

(d) Chronic hallucinations

II. Course criterion

A final decision about diagnosis cannot be made before a follow-up period of at least five years has shown a chronic course of disease.

Based on: Langfeldt, G. (1969) Schizophrenia: diagnosis and prognosis. *Behav. Science*, **14**, 173–82.

COMMENTARY

Ever since his somatic studies of schizophrenia in the years 1923–1926, Langfeldt, following Kraepelin's footsteps, has stressed the significance of restricting the diagnosis of schizophrenia to a group of disorders which, as proven by individual follow-up investigations, have a poor prognosis.

Langfeldt's prognostic factors have been derived from two follow-up studies, the first (Langfeldt, 1937, 1939) carried through at a time when somatic treatment wasn't yet available, the second (Langfeldt, 1956) after introduction of shock-treatment and lobotomy. The following are considered by Langfeldt (1956) as unfavorable prognostic factors:

a. An emotionally and intellectually poorly developed premorbid personality
b. No demonstrable precipitating factors
c. Insidious onset
d. A symptomatology mainly characteristic of Kraepelin's dementia praecox with the basic traits of autism and emotional blunting as stressed especially by Eugen Bleuler (1911) in his description of the basic traits in schizophrenia. Particularly unfavorable are those cases characterized by typical depersonalization and derealization symptoms with clear consciousness and the absence of admixtures from other psychoses
e. An unfavorable environment before and after the outbreak of the disease

Langfeldt's (1969) diagnostic criteria for schizophrenia are part of the prognostic factors (symptoms of d) which were derived statistically, and Langfeldt himself states that 'in the single case it is the constellation of the different signs and symptoms, which indicates the further course.' His diagnostic criteria were reformulated and appear in their latest version in his papers in 1960 and 1969. They enable us to differentiate between two groups of 'psychoses usually diagnosed as schizophrenia' (Langfeldt): a nuclear group with poor prognosis (which he labeled 'genuine types of schizophrenia' and a second group characterized by a schizophrenia-like picture but lacking in poor prognosis symptomatology (which he labeled 'schizophreniform psychoses,' a term which does not represent a diagnostic entity).

This differentiation at that time was important for therapeutic considerations: in his follow-up studies Langfeldt found that the course of poor prognosis schizophrenia was uninfluenced by somatic therapy and that of schizophreniform disorder in many cases was better with somatic (especially insulin-coma) treatment than it was before the advent of somatic treatment.

The symptomatological criteria can be divided into inclusion and exclusion criteria: the inclusion criteria consist on the one hand of observed symptoms and on the other hand of reported symptoms. Exclusion criteria are observed or reported symptoms of organic brain disorder, infection, or intoxication. Non-symptomatological criteria concern a five-year observation period for a final decision of diagnosis (II).

Langfeldt's (1969) criteria Ia–d are only 'significant clues to a diagnosis of schizophrenia' and a final decision can only be made after five years of individual follow-up. Langfeldt does not specify whether criteria other than those important for prognosis are considered by him for diagnosing schizophrenia. He merely applies his diagnostic criteria to patients already diagnosed as schizophrenic by other classificatory systems ('psychoses usually diagnosed as schizophrenia').

Of great importance is the differential diagnosis to schizophreniform disorder, a heterogeneous group of disorders characterized by a 'schizophrenia-like symptomatology' but without the symptoms of the poor prognosis group. Compared with schizophrenia, schizophreniform disorders have a much better prognosis. The following factors are considered by Langfeldt (1956) to be correlated with good prognosis:

a. An emotionally and intellectually well-developed premorbid personality
b. Demonstrable precipitating factors
c. Acute onset
d. A symptomatology characterized by a mixed picture, especially with admixtures of manic-depressive traits, cloudiness or symptoms of organic (perhaps toxic) and psychogenic origin, and lacking the typical blunting of emotional life
e. A favorable environment before and after the outbreak of the disorder, with a psychologically correct attitude on the part of the surroundings to the problems of the patient

Langfeldt's diagnostic criteria for schizophrenia are derived from his 'poor-prognosis' factors and therefore restrict the diagnosis of schizophrenia to a poor-prognosis group. Brockington *et al.* (1978) found a good interrater reliability for these criteria and highly significant associations with clinical state and social breakdown. (These authors used only part 1 of Langfeldt's criteria.) Despite their success in predicting poor prognosis, Langfeldt's criteria are unsatisfactory by contemporary standards, because the groups of symptoms that he regards as characteristic of schizophrenia are not defined with adequate clarity (Kendell *et al.*, 1979).

An interesting attempt to bring Langfeldt's criteria nearer to modern standards of research criteria was carried through by Landmark (1982), who rearranged Langfeldt's system for clinical as well as statistical purposes (under Langfeldt's own supervision).

B5

International classification of diseases (ICD), 8th and 9th revisions

Psychoses (290–299)

Psychosis includes those conditions in which impairment of mental functions has developed to a degree that interferes grossly with insight, ability to meet some of the ordinary demands of life, or adequate contact with reality. It is not an exact or well-defined term. Mental retardation is excluded (310–315).

295. Schizophrenic psychoses

A group of psychoses in which there is a fundamental disturbance of personality, a characteristic distortion of thinking, often a sense of being controlled by alien forces, delusions which may be bizarre, disturbed perception, abnormal affect out of keeping with the real situation, and autism. Nevertheless, clear consciousness and intellectual capacity are usually maintained. The disturbance of personality involves its most basic functions which give the normal person his feeling of individuality, uniqueness and self-direction. The most intimate thoughts, feelings and acts are often felt to be known to or shared by others and explanatory delusions may develop, to the effect that natural or supernatural forces are at work to influence the schizophrenic person's thoughts and actions in ways that are often bizarre. He may see himself as the pivot of all that happens. Hallucinations, especially of hearing, are common and may comment on the patient or address him. Perception is frequently

Sources of criteria: ICD 8th Revision (1967) *WHO manual of the international statistical classification of diseases V* (1965 revision). Geneva: WHO. ICD 9th Revision (1978) *Mental disorders: glossary and guide to their classification in accordance with the ninth revision of the international classification of diseases.* Geneva: WHO.

disturbed in other ways; there may be perplexity, irrelevant features may become all-important and, accompanied by passivity feelings, may lead the patient to believe that everyday objects and situations possess a special, usually sinister, meaning intended for him. In the characteristic schizophrenic disturbance of thinking, peripheral and irrelevant features of a total concept, which are inhibited in normal directed mental activity, are brought to the forefront and utilized in place of the elements relevant and appropriate to the situation. Thus thinking becomes vague, elliptical and obscure, and its expression in speech sometimes incomprehensible. Breaks and interpolations in the flow of consecutive thought are frequent, and the patient may be convinced that his thoughts are being withdrawn by some outside agency. Mood may be shallow, capricious or incongruous. Ambivalence and disturbance of volition may appear as inertia, negativism or stupor. Catatonia may be present. The diagnosis 'schizophrenia' should not be made unless there is, or has been evident during the same illness, characteristic disturbance of thought, perception, mood, conduct, or personality – preferably in at least two of these areas. The diagnosis should not be restricted to conditions running a protracted, deteriorating, or chronic course. In addition to making the diagnosis on the criteria just given, effort should be made to specify one of the following subdivisions of schizophrenia, according to the predominant symptoms.

Includes: schizophrenia of the types described in 295.0–295.9 occurring in children
Excludes: childhood-type schizophrenia (299.9)
            infantile autism (299.0)

295.0 Simple type

A psychosis in which there is insidious development of oddities of conduct, inability to meet the demands of society, and decline in total performance. Delusions and hallucinations are not in evidence and the condition is less obviously psychotic than are the hebephrenic, catatonic and paranoid types of schizophrenia. With increasing social impoverishment vagrancy may ensue and the patient becomes self-absorbed, idle and aimless. Because the schizophrenic symptoms are not clear-cut, diagnosis of this form should be made sparingly, if at all.

Schizophrenia simplex
Excludes: latent schizophrenia (295.5)

295.1 Hebephrenic type

A form of schizophrenia in which affective changes are prominent, delusions and hallucinations fleeting and fragmentary, behaviour irresponsible and unpredictable and mannerisms common. The mood is shallow and inappropriate, accompanied by giggling or self-satisfied, self-absorbed smiling, or by a lofty manner, grimaces, mannerisms, pranks, hypochondriacal complaints and reiterated phrases. Thought is disorganized. There is a tendency to remain solitary, and behaviour seems empty of purpose and feeling. This form of schizophrenia usually starts between the ages of 15 and 25 years.

Hebephrenia

295.2 Catatonic type

Includes as an essential feature prominent psychomotor disturbances often alternating between extremes such as hyperkinesis and stupor, or automatic obedience and negativism. Constrained attitudes may be maintained for long periods: if the patients' limbs are put in some unnatural position they may be held there for some time after the external force has been removed. Severe excitement may be a striking feature of the condition. Depressive or hypomanic concomitants may be present.

Catatonic:	Schizophrenic:
agitation	catalepsy
excitation	catatonia
stupor	flexibilitas cerea

295.3 Paranoid type

The form of schizophrenia in which relatively stable delusions, which may be accompanied by hallucinations dominate the clinical picture. The delusions are frequently of persecution but may take other forms (for example of jealousy, exalted birth, Messianic mission, or bodily change). Hallucinations and erratic behaviour may occur; in some cases conduct is seriously disturbed from the outset, thought disorder may be gross, and affective flattening with fragmentary delusions and hallucinations may develop.

Paraphrenic schizophrenia
Excludes: paraphrenia, involutional paranoid state (297.2)
paranoia (297.1)

295.4 Acute schizophrenic episode

Schizophrenic disorders, other than those listed above, in which there is a dream-like state with slight clouding of consciousness and perplexity. External things, people and events may become charged with personal significance for the patient. There may be ideas of reference and emotional turmoil. In many such cases remission occurs within a few weeks or months, even without treatment.

Oneirophrenia   Schizophreniform:
                 attack
                 psychosis, confusional type

Excludes: acute forms of schizophrenia of:
            catatonic type (295.2)
            hebephrenic type (295.1)
            paranoid type (295.3)
            simple type (295.0)

295.5 Latent schizophrenia

It has not been possible to produce a generally acceptable description for this condition. It is not recommended for general use, but a description is provided for those who believe it to be useful: a condition of eccentric or inconsequent behaviour and anomalies of affect which give the impression of schizophrenia though no definite and characteristic schizophrenic anomalies, present or past, have been manifest. The inclusion terms indicate that this is the best place to classify some other poorly defined varieties of schizophrenia.

Latent schizophrenic reaction   Schizophrenia:
Schizophrenia: pseudoneurotic
    borderline   pseudopsychopathic
    prepsychotic
    prodromal

Excludes: schizoid personality (301.2)

295.6 Residual schizophrenia

A chronic form of schizophrenia in which the symptoms that persist from the acute phase have mostly lost their sharpness. Emotional response is blunted and thought disorder, even when gross, does not prevent the accomplishment of routine work.

Chronic undifferentiated schizophrenia
Restzustand (schizophrenic)
Schizophrenic residual state

295.7 Schizoaffective type

A psychosis in which pronounced manic or depressive features are intermingled with schizophrenic features and which tends towards remission without permanent defect, but which is prone to recur. The diagnosis should be made only when both the affective and schizophrenic symptoms are pronounced.

Cyclic schizophrenia
Mixed schizophrenic and affective psychosis

Schizoaffective psychosis
Schizophreniform psychosis, affective type

295.8 Other

Schizophrenia of specified type not classifiable under 295.0–295.7.

Acute (undifferentiated)   Atypical schizophrenia
   schizophrenia   Coenesthopathic
                                     schizophrenia

Excludes: infantile autism (299.0)

295.9 Unspecified

To be used only as a last resort.

Schizophrenia NOS*
Schizophrenic reaction NOS
Schizophreniform psychosis NOS

* Editor's note: Not otherwise specified (NOS).

COMMENTARY

International efforts for establishing joint classifications of illnesses began toward the end of the last century. The World Health Organization (WHO) has assumed these efforts since 1948. The International Classification of Diseases, Injuries, and Causes of Death (ICD) is the result. Its fifth chapter is devoted to psychiatric illnesses. As of the 8th revision (1967), schizophrenic disorders bear the code number 295; subgroups are classified by means of a fourth digit into ten entities (295.0–295.9). The 9th revision (1978) corresponds to the 8th in this respect, so that both can be presented together. One difference is that the international glossary (Glossary, 1974), which already existed at the time of the 8th revision and had been incorporated into the German publication of the Deutsche Gesellschaft für Psychiatrie und Nervenheilkunde (German Association of Psychiatry and Neurology [DGPN]), was not incorporated into the original English publication of the 8th revision by the WHO. This glossary is now a part of the diagnostic schema in the 9th edition. The ICD's purpose is to achieve an internationally utilizable instrument of classification. In order to attain this goal, compromises had to be made. The glossary's integration should reduce the risk of unreliable application.

Schizophrenia (295) in the ICD is classified among the psychoses; that is, among illnesses 'in which impairment of mental functions has developed to a degree that interferes grossly with insight, ability to meet some of the ordinary demands of life, or adequate contact with reality' (ICD 9th revision, p. 19). In order to meet the criteria, then, the characteristic disorder must present a certain degree of severity. Schizophrenia is defined as 'a group of psychoses in which there is a

fundamental disturbance of personality,
a characteristic distortion of thinking,
often a sense of feeling controlled by alien forces,
delusions that may be bizarre,
disturbed perception,
abnormal affect which is out of keeping with the real situation, and
autism' (ICD 9th revision, pp. 26–27).

'Nevertheless clear consciousness and intellectual capacity are usually maintained' (ICD 9th revision, p. 27).

(Bleuler's concept of schizophrenia clearly influenced these definitions. See Chapter B2 for a comparison with his criteria) 'The diagnosis "schizophrenia" should not be made unless there is, or has been evident during the same illness, characteristic disturbances of thought, perception, mood, conduct, or personality – preferably in at least two of these areas.' (ICD 9th revision, p. 27). On the other hand non-symptomatological criteria, especially concerning illness course, are not to be considered for classification. This concept of schizophrenia is thus a broad one, based partly on symptomatology and partly on the degree (psychotic) of severity. Its position between organic and affective psychoses reflects traditional hierarchical assumptions. The symptoms concerned reflect in part disturbances of experience and in part disturbances of behavior, gathered partly from the patient's reports and partly from the patient's behavior.

The fourth-digit order concerns the identification of subgroups. Its application is facilitated by more or less precise descriptions and a listing of syndromatological notions for subgroup inclusion and/or exclusion. Above all this is of consequence for the delimitation of paranoid schizophrenia from other paranoid psychoses (ICD 297) and the delimitation of latent schizophrenia from schizoid personality (ICD 301.2). Criteria other than symptomatological ones appear in the description of the subgroups, especially those to do with illness chronology. These can refer on the one hand to the form the illness presented at onset or during its course, or on the other hand to the age of predilection:

295.0 Simple type	Insidious onset
295.1 Hebephrenic type	Onset mainly between the ages of 15 and 25 years
295.3 Paranoid type	Relatively stable
295.4 Acute schizophrenic episode	Acute onset, remission mostly within a few weeks or months

295.6 Residual schizophrenia	Chronic form following acute episodes
295.7 Schizoaffective type	Remission without permanent defect

Such indications, however, are not systematically offered. As a rule, *all subgroups are syndromatological*. This applies also to 295.4 acute schizophrenic episode; its description does contain illness course criteria (acute onset, remission), but it is above all characterized by its psychopathological features in cross-sectional presentation.

The ICD concept of schizophrenia reflects the broadest and most generally disseminated teaching of schizophrenic psychoses. This classic concept is based on descriptive psychopathology and characteristic disturbances of basic psychic functioning. A certain degree of symptom intensity is required. The possibility of establishing operational criteria is at best meager. It is valid in the absence of organicity. Schizophrenic symptoms take precedence over affective ones for diagnostic purposes (from whence the rubric schizoaffective type) and remain valid on the sole condition that they once manifested themselves. Evolutional and etiopathogenetic considerations beyond the exclusion of organic origin are ignored; the former do appear unsystematically in the subgroups. The recommendation to apply the concept only when the presence of at least two of the characteristic symptoms is confirmed is an attempt to increase the validity of the concept by limiting its application.

As early as 1975, Helmchen reviewed the ICD diagnostic concepts of schizophrenia. He investigated to what extent they conformed to five 'axial' criteria (symptomatology, time, etiology, intensity, certainty) and made practical recommendations for their improvement along this line. The schizophrenia concept of the 8th and 9th revisions of the ICD tends to move in the direction of such multiaxiality, but so far there are no signs of systematic involvement.

The ICD concept of schizophrenia is officially used by UN member nations, making it one of the concepts presently enjoying the greatest dissemination. If one considers it practically identical with Bleuler's (1911) traditional concept, it probably is the most widespread. It presents a store of relatively well-elaborated psychopathological criteria of limited etiological validity covering an area of functional psychoses. Thanks to the incorporation of a glossary, chances for the 9th revision's reliable application look promising.

B6

International classification of diseases (ICD), 1989 draft for the 10th revision

CRITERIA

F20–F29 Schizophrenia, schizotypal and delusional disorders

Schizophrenia is the commonest and most important member of this group. Schizotypal disorder possesses many of the characteristic features of schizophrenic disorders and is probably genetically related to them, but this disorder does not exhibit the hallucinations, delusions, and gross behavioral disturbances of schizophrenia itself, and so does not always come to medical attention. Most of the delusional disorders are probably unrelated to schizophrenia though they may be difficult to distinguish clinically, particularly in their early stages. They are a heterogeneous and ill-understood collection of disorders which can conveniently be divided by their typical duration into a group of persistent delusional disorders and a larger group of acute and transient psychotic disorders. The latter appear to be particularly common in developing countries. The sub-divisions listed here should be regarded as provisional. Schizoaffective disorders have been retained in this section in spite of their controversial nature.

F20 Schizophrenia

The schizophrenic disorders are characterized in general by fundamental and characteristic distortions of thinking and perception, and affects that are inappropriate or blunted. Clear consciousness and intellectual capacity are usually maintained although certain cognitive deficits may evolve in the course of time. The disturbance involves the most basic

Source of criteria: ICD–10 (1989a) 1989 Draft of Chapter V, categories F00–F99 / mental and behavioral disorders. Clinical descriptions and diagnostic guidelines. April 1989. Division of Mental Health, Geneva: WHO.

functions which give the normal person a feeling of individuality, unique-ness and self-direction. The most intimate thoughts, feelings and acts are often felt to be known to or shared by others and explanatory delusions may develop, to the effect that natural or supernatural forces are at work to influence the afflicted individual's thoughts and actions in ways that are often bizarre. They may see themselves as the pivot of all that happens. Hallucinations, especially auditory, are common and may comment on the subject's behavior or thoughts. Perception is frequently disturbed in other ways: colors or sounds may seem unduly vivid or altered in quality and irrelevant features of ordinary things may appear more important than the whole object or situation. Perplexity is also common early on and frequently leads to a belief that everyday situations possess a special, usually sinister, meaning intended uniquely for the individual. In the characteristic schizophrenic disturbance of thinking, peripheral and irrel-evant features of a total concept, which are inhibited in normal directed mental activity, are brought to the forefront and utilized in place of those which are relevant and appropriate to the situation. Thus thinking becomes vague, elliptical and obscure, and its expression in speech sometimes incomprehensible. Breaks and interpolations in the train of thought are frequent, and thoughts may seem to be withdrawn by some outside agency. Mood is characteristically shallow, capricious or incon-gruous. Ambivalence and disturbance of volition may appear as inertia, negativism or stupor. Catatonia may be present. The onset may be acute with seriously disturbed behavior, or insidious, with a gradual develop-ment of odd ideas and conduct. The course shows equally great variation and is by no means inevitably chronic or deteriorating (the course is specified by fifth character categories). In a proportion of cases, which may vary in different cultures and populations, the outcome is complete, or nearly complete, recovery. The sexes are approximately equally affected but the onset tends to be later in women.

Although no strictly pathognomonic symptoms can be identified, for practical purposes it is useful to divide the above symptoms into two groups which have special importance for the diagnosis, and often occur together, such as:

(i) thought echo, thought insertion or withdrawal, and thought broad-casting;

(ii) delusions of control, influence or passivity, clearly referred to body or limb movements or specific thoughts, actions, or sensations; and delusional perception;

(iii) hallucinatory voices giving a running commentary on the patient's behavior, or discussing him between themselves, or other types of hallucinatory voices coming from some part of the body;

(iv) persistent delusions of other kinds that are culturally inappropriate and implausible, such as religious or political identity, superhuman powers and abilities, etc.;

(v) persistent hallucinations in any modality, when accompanied by either fleeting or half-formed delusions without clear affective content, or by persistent over-valued ideas, or when occurring every day for weeks or months on end;

(vi) breaks or interpolations in the train of thought, resulting in incoherence or irrelevant speech, or neologisms;

(vii) catatonic behavior, such as excitement, posturing or waxy flexibility, negativism, mutism and stupor;

(viii) 'negative' symptoms such as marked apathy, paucity of speech, and blunting or incongruity of emotional responses (these usually result in social withdrawal and lowering of social performance). It must be clear that these are not due to depression or to neuroleptic medication.

Diagnostic guidelines

The normal requirement for a diagnosis of schizophrenia is that a minimum of one very clear symptom (and usually two or more if less clear-cut) belonging to any one of the groups listed as (i) to (iv) above, or symptoms from at least two of the groups referred to as (v) to (viii), should have been clearly present for most of the time during a period of one month or more. Conditions meeting such symptomatic requirements but of a duration less than one month (whether treated or not) should be diagnosed in the first instance as acute schizophrenia-like psychotic disorder (F23.2) and reclassified as schizophrenia if the symptoms persist for longer periods of time.

Viewed retrospectively it may be clear that a prodromal phase in which symptoms and behavior, such as loss of interest in work, social activities and personal appearance and hygiene, together with generalized anxiety and mild degrees of depression and preoccupation may precede the onset of psychotic symptoms by weeks or even months. Because of the difficulty in timing onset, the one-month duration criterion applies only to specific symptoms listed above and not to any prodromal non-psychotic phase.

The diagnosis of schizophrenia should not be made in the presence of extensive depressive or manic symptoms unless it is clear that schizophrenic symptoms antedated the affective disturbance. If both schizophrenic and affective symptoms develop together and are evenly balanced then the diagnosis of schizoaffective disorder (F25) should be made, even if the schizophrenic symptoms by themselves would have justified the diagnosis of schizophrenia. Nor should schizophrenia be diagnosed in the presence of overt brain disease or during states of drug intoxication or withdrawal. Similar disorders developing in the presence of epilepsy or other brain disease should be coded under F06.2, and those induced by drugs under F1x.5.

Pattern of course

The course of schizophrenic disorders can be classified by using the following fifth character codes:

F20.x0   continuous
F20.x1   episodic with progressive deficit
F20.x2   episodic with stable deficit
F20.x3   episodic remittent
F20.x4   incomplete remission
F20.x5   complete remission
F20.x8   other
F20.x9   period of observation less than one year

F20.0   Paranoid schizophrenia

This is the commonest type of schizophrenia in most parts of the world. The clinical picture is dominated by relatively stable delusions, usually accompanied by hallucinations, particularly of the auditory variety. Disturbances of affect, volition and speech, and catatonic symptoms, are not prominent.

The most prominent manifestations are paranoid delusions and hallucinations (the paranoid-hallucinatory syndrome):

(i) abnormal subjective experiences such as thought echo, insertion or withdrawal and thought broadcasting;
(ii) disturbances of the perception of time, space, colour, visual form, body image, etc.;
(iii) delusions of control, influence or passivity;
(iv) auditory hallucinations often taking the form of a commentary on thoughts or actions, or voices discussing the subject between themselves.

Other common symptoms include:

(v) delusions of persecution, reference, jealousy, exalted birth, special mission or bodily change;
(vi) hallucinatory voices speaking to the subject, threatening him, abusing him or giving him commands, or auditory hallucinations without any verbal form, e.g. whistling, humming or laughing;
(vii) hallucinations of smell or taste, or sexual or other bodily sensation; visual hallucinations may also occur but are rarely predominant;
(viii) thought disorder can be gross in the acute state but often delusions and hallucinations are described with clarity;
(ix) affect is usually less blunted than in other forms but a minor degree of incongruity is common, as are moods such as irritability, anger, fear, and suspicion;

(x) 'negative' symptoms such as blunting of affect and impaired volition are often present but do not dominate the clinical picture.

The course of paranoid schizophrenia may be episodic, with partial or complete remissions, or chronic. In the latter variety the florid symptoms persist over years and it is difficult to distinguish discrete episodes. The onset tends to be later than in the hebephrenic and catatonic forms.

Diagnostic guidelines

The various types of schizophrenia are not sharply demarcated from one another and patients may change from one type to another in the course of their illness. The general criteria for a diagnosis of schizophrenia (see F20 above) must be satisfied. In addition hallucinations and/or delusions must be prominent, and disturbances of affect, volition and speech, and catatonic symptoms, relatively inconspicuous. Normally the hallucinations will be of the kind described in (iv), (vi) and (vii) above. The delusions can be of almost any kind but delusions of control, influence or passivity, and persecutory beliefs of various kinds, are the most characteristic.

In differential diagnosis it is important to exclude epileptic and drug-induced psychoses, and to remember that persecutory delusions might carry little diagnostic weight in people from certain countries or cultures.

Includes: paraphrenic schizophrenia.

F20.1 Hebephrenic schizophrenia

A form of schizophrenia in which affective changes are prominent, delusions and hallucinations fleeting and fragmentary, behavior irresponsible and unpredictable, and mannerisms common. The mood is shallow and inappropriate and often accompanied by giggling or self-satisfied, self-absorbed smiling, or by a lofty manner, grimaces, mannerisms, pranks, hypochondriacal complaints and reiterated phrases. Thought is disorganized, and speech rambling and incoherent. There is a tendency to remain solitary, and behavior seems empty of purpose and feeling. This form of schizophrenia usually starts between the ages of 15 and 25 years and tends to have a poor prognosis because of the rapid development of 'negative' symptoms, particularly flattening of affect and loss of volition.

In addition disturbances of affect and volition, and thought disorder, should be prominent. Hallucinations and delusions may be present but should not be prominent. Drive and determination are lost and goals abandoned, so that the patient's behavior becomes characteristically aimless and empty of purpose. A superficial and manneristic preoccupation with religion, philosophy and other abstract themes may add to the listener's difficulty in following the train of thought.

Diagnostic guidelines

The general criteria for a diagnosis of schizophrenia (see F20 above) must be satisfied. Hebephrenia should normally only be diagnosed in adolescents or young adults. The premorbid personality is characteristically, but not necessarily, rather shy and solitary. For a confident diagnosis of hebephrenia a period of two or three months of continuous observation is usually necessary, in order to ensure that the characteristic behaviors described above are sustained.

Includes: disorganized schizophrenia.

F20.2 Catatonic schizophrenia

Prominent psychomotor disturbances are an essential and dominant feature and may alternate between extremes such as hyperkinesis and stupor, or automatic obedience and negativism. Constrained attitudes and postures may be maintained for long periods. Episodes of violent excitement may be a striking feature of the condition.

For reasons which are ill-understood catatonic schizophrenia is now rarely seen in industrial countries, though it remains common elsewhere. These catatonic phenomena may be combined with a dream-like (oneiroid) state with vivid scenic hallucinations.

Diagnostic guidelines

The general criteria for a diagnosis of schizophrenia (F20 above) must be satisfied. Isolated catatonic symptoms may occur transitorily in the context of any other subtype of schizophrenia. For a diagnosis of catatonic schizophrenia one or more of the following behaviors, or any sequence of them, should dominate the clinical picture: (i) stupor (marked decrease in reactivity to the environment and reduction of spontaneous movements and activity) or mutism; (ii) excitement (apparently purposeless motor activity, not influenced by external stimuli); (iii) posturing (voluntary assumption and maintenance of inappropriate or bizarre postures); (iv) negativism (an apparently motiveless resistance to all instructions or attempts to be moved or movement in the opposite direction); (v) rigidity (maintenance of a rigid posture against efforts to be moved); (vi) waxy flexibility (maintenance of limbs and body in externally imposed positions); and (vii) other symptoms such as command automatism (automatic compliance with instructions), and perseveration of words and phrases.

In uncommunicative subjects with behavioral manifestations of catatonic disorder the diagnosis of schizophrenia may have to be provisional until adequate evidence of the presence of other symptoms is obtained. It is also vital to appreciate that catatonic symptoms are not diagnostic of schizophrenia. A catatonic symptom or symptoms may also be provoked by brain disease or metabolic disturbances or alcohol and drugs and may also occur in mood disorders.

Includes: schizophrenic catalepsy; schizophrenic catatonia; schizophrenic flexibilitas cerea.

F20.3 Undifferentiated schizophrenia

Conditions meeting the general diagnostic criteria for schizophrenia (see F20 above) but not conforming to any of the above subtypes, or exhibiting the features of more than one of them without a clear predominance of a particular set of diagnostic characteristics. This rubric should only be used for psychotic conditions (i.e. residual schizophrenia and post-schizophrenic depression are excluded), and after an attempt has been made to classify the condition into one of the three preceding categories.

Diagnostic guidelines

This subtype should be reserved for patients who: (i) meet the diagnostic criteria for schizophrenia; (ii) do not satisfy the criteria for the paranoid, hebephrenic, or catatonic subtypes; (iii) do not satisfy the criteria for residual schizophrenia or post-schizophrenic depression.

Includes: atypical schizophrenia.

F20.4 Post-schizophrenic depression

A depressive episode, which may be prolonged, arising in the aftermath of a schizophrenic illness. Some schizophrenic symptoms must still be present but they no longer dominate the clinical picture. These persisting schizophrenic symptoms may be 'positive' or 'negative' though the latter are most common. It is uncertain, and immaterial to the diagnosis, to what extent the depressive symptoms have merely been uncovered by the resolution of earlier psychotic symptoms rather than being a new development, or to what extent they are an intrinsic part of schizophrenia rather than a psychological reaction to it. They are rarely sufficiently severe or extensive to meet criteria for a severe depressive episode (F32.2 and .3) and it is often difficult to decide which of the patient's symptoms are due to depression and which to neuroleptic medication or to the impaired volition and affective flattening of schizophrenia itself. This depressive disorder is associated with an increased risk of suicide.

Diagnostic guidelines

The diagnosis should only be made if: (i) the patient has had a schizophrenic illness meeting the general criteria for schizophrenia (F20) within the past twelve months; (ii) some schizophrenic symptoms are still present; and (iii) the depressive symptoms are prominent and distressing, fulfilling at least the criteria for a depressive episode (F32.—) and have been present for at least two weeks. If the patient no longer has any schizophrenic symptoms a depressive episode should be diagnosed (F32). If schizophrenic symptoms are still florid and prominent the diagnosis should remain that of the appropriate schizophrenic subtype (F20.0, F20.1, F20.2, or F20.3).

F20.5 Residual schizophrenia

A chronic stage in the development of a schizophrenic illness in which there has been a clear progression from an early stage (comprising one or more episodes with psychotic symptoms meeting the general criteria for schizophrenia described above) to a later state characterized by long-term, though not necessarily irreversible, 'negative' symptoms and impairments.

Diagnostic guidelines

For a confident diagnosis, the following requirements should be met: (i) prominent 'negative' schizophrenic symptoms i.e. psychomotor slowing; underactivity; blunting of affect; passivity and lack of initiative; poverty of quantity or content of speech; poor non-verbal communication by facial expression, eye contact, voice modulation and posture; poor self-care and social performance; (ii) evidence in the past of at least one clear-cut psychotic episode meeting the diagnostic criteria for schizophrenia; (iii) a period of *at least one year* during which the intensity and frequency of florid symptoms such as delusions and hallucinations have been minimal or substantially reduced *and* the 'negative' schizophrenic syndrome has been present; (iv) absence of dementia or other organic brain pathology; absence of chronic depression or institutionalism sufficient to explain the negative impairments.

If adequate information about the patient's previous history cannot be obtained, and it therefore cannot be established that criteria for schizophrenia have been met at some time in the past, it may be necessary to make a provisional diagnosis of residual schizophrenia.

Includes: chronic undifferentiated schizophrenia; 'Restzustand'; schizophrenic residual state.

F20.6 Simple schizophrenia

An uncommon disorder in which there is an insidious but progressive development of oddities of conduct, inability to meet the demands of society, and decline in total performance. Delusions and hallucinations are not in evidence, and the disorder is less obviously psychotic than the hebephrenic and catatonic types of schizophrenia. The characteristic 'negative' features of residual schizophrenia (e.g. blunting of affect, loss of volition, etc.) develop without being preceded by any overt psychotic symptoms. With increasing social impoverishment vagrancy may ensue and the subject becomes self-absorbed, idle and aimless.

Diagnostic guidelines

Simple schizophrenia is a difficult diagnosis to make with any confidence because it depends on establishing the slowly progressive development of the characteristic 'negative' symptoms of residual schizophrenia (see F20.5 above) without any history of hallucinations, delusions, or other manifestations of an earlier psychotic episode.

Includes: schizophrenia simplex.

F20.8 Other schizophrenia

Includes: coenesthopathic schizophrenia.
Excludes: acute schizophrenia (F23.2); cyclic schizophrenia (F25.2); latent schizophrenia (F23.3).

F20.9 Schizophrenia, unspecified

F21 Schizotypal disorder

A disorder characterized by eccentric behavior and anomalies of thinking and affect which resemble those seen in schizophrenia, though no definite and characteristic schizophrenic anomalies have occurred at any stage. There is no dominant or typical disturbance but any of the following may be present: (i) an affect which is cold and aloof, and often accompanied by anhedonia; (ii) behavior or appearance which is odd, eccentric or peculiar; (iii) poor rapport with others and a tendency to social withdrawal; (iv) ideas of reference, paranoid ideas, or bizarre, fantastic beliefs and autistic preoccupations not amounting to true delusions; (v) obsessive rumi-nations without inner resistance, often with dysmorphophobic, sexual, or aggressive contents; (vi) occasional somatosensory illusions and deper-sonalization or derealization experiences; (vii) vague, circumstantial, metaphorical, overelaborate, and often stereotyped thinking and speech, without gross incoherence or irrelevance; (viii) occasional transient quasi-psychotic episodes with intense illusions, auditory or other hallucinations, and delusion-like ideas, usually occurring without external provocation.

The disorder runs a chronic course with fluctuations of intensity. Occasionally it evolves into overt schizophrenia. There is no definite onset and its evolution and course are usually those of a personality disorder. It is more common in individuals genetically related to schizophrenics and is believed to be part of the genetic 'spectrum' of schizophrenia.

Diagnostic guidelines

This diagnostic rubric is not recommended for general use because it is not clearly demarcated either from simple schizophrenia or from schizoid or paranoid personality disorders. If the term is used, three or four of the typical features listed above should have been present, continuously or episodically, for *at least two years*. The subject must never have met criteria for schizophrenia itself. A history of schizophrenia in a first-degree relative gives additional weight to the diagnosis but is not a prerequisite.

Includes: latent schizophrenia; latent schizophrenic reaction; borderline schizophrenia; prepsychotic schizophrenia; prodromal schizophrenia; pseudoneurotic schizophrenia; pseudopsychopathic schizophrenia; schizotypal personality disorder.

Excludes: schizoid personality disorder (F60.1); Asperger's syndrome (F84.5).

COMMENTARY

During the last few years the Division of Mental Health of the World Health Organization (WHO) has been preparing the 10th revision of the fifth chapter of the International Classification of Diseases (ICD), which traditionally contains the 'Mental and behavioral disorders.' For this purpose the psychiatric world, especially the World Psychiatric Association (WPA), has been broadly consulted. The draft now exists in a form (ICD–10, April 1989*a* draft) that will probably not undergo any further important modifications before the resolution on the 10th revision is passed.

In contrast to the 9th revision (ICD–9), the 1989 draft for the 10th revision is arranged in an alphanumeric system of codes, in which the fifth chapter 'Mental and Developmental Disorders' occupies the categories F00–F99. This series of categories comprises sections which group together, at least on the basis of hypothetical affiliation, disorders which were assigned to separate categories in ICD–9. (Instead, other combinations of categories in ICD–9, above all the organization of the whole system according to psychoses and other disorders, have been abandoned).

The section F2, with the codes F20–F29, comprises **schizophrenia**, **schizotypal**, and **delusional disorders**, namely:

F20 Schizophrenia
F21 Schizotypal disorder
F22 Persistent delusional disorders (see E5)
F23 Acute and transient psychotic disorders
F24 Induced delusional disorders (see E5)
F25 Schizoaffective disorders (see D4)

F28 Other non-organic psychotic disorders
F29 Non-organic psychosis, not otherwise specified

This section lies between the two sections dealing with organic mental disorders (F00–F09, F10–F19) and the section on **mood (affective) disorders** (F30–F39). It contains disorders that ICD–9 assigned to schizophrenic psychoses (295) and paranoid psychoses (297, 298.3, 298.4) in a different arrangement (see Chapters B5 and E4). All disorders that were allocated to schizophrenic psychoses (295) in ICD–9 can be found in this section, albeit only in part under F20, schizophrenia.

The ICD–10 drafts which have been presented thus far contain comprehensive descriptions and diagnostic guidelines for each category in this chapter, and they also provide equivalent terms for diagnostic attribution which they do not employ. The ICD–10 drafts surpass ICD-9 not only in the number of diagnostic concepts, but also in the amount of information provided for them.

The fifth chapter of the 10th revision is being developed in several versions. We are referring to: (1) The version 'for general clinical, educational and service use' with the title *Clinical descriptions and diagnostic guidelines* (ICD–10, 1989*a*); (2) a set of diagnostic criteria for research (ICD–10, 1989*b*). To be developed later and examined in field studies are: (a) a multiaspect system for the description of patients and their disorders; (b) a simplified form for use in primary health care; (c) a short glossary as part of the complete ICD–10 revision.

The general description of schizophrenic psychoses in the 'clinical descriptions and diagnostic guidelines' closely resembles that in the ICD–9 glossary (see Chapter B5). From it, however, eight groups of symptoms are derived and especially emphasized (i to viii). i to iii correspond to first rank symptoms of Kurt Schneider, and so to phenomena of experience (see Chapter B3); alternatively, i to vi represent so-called positive symptoms, vii catatonic psychomotor disturbances, and viii so-called negative symptoms (preponderantly phenomena of expression).

More attention is given to ensuring the diagnosis in the diagnostic guidelines than in ICD–9. There is a fourfold provision for this security:

From the symptom groups i to iv there should be at least one clear symptom *or* from at least two of the symptom groups v to viii symptoms present in order to make the diagnosis. A similar, although less defined proposal, may also be found in ICD–9.

The diagnosis should be considered only for disorders that last for at least one month, disregarding prodromes; for a shorter period a diagnosis from the F23 category, acute and transient psychotic disorders, should be made provisionally. ICD–9 did not explicitly recognize a time criterion as a restriction of the schizophrenia concept. The time criterion employed in the ICD–10 draft is not identical with that of

DSM–III and DSM–III–R (see Chapters B9 and B10). It refers explicitly not to the entire course of a symptomatologically recognizable period of illness, even though prodromal symptoms may only temporarily contribute, but to the fully developed psychosis alone. (Fifth character codes describe the entire course in terms of its chronicity [continuous] or intermittence with different episode outcomes, on condition that the course of the disorder lasts at least one year. Therefore, a greater degree of both diagnostic certainty and information for the total diagnostic concept may be attained through a certain duration of the full-blown psychosis and the introduction of reference numbers describing the course. Contrasting a simple, chronic course [continuous] and different outcomes of episodic courses prompts a discriminating consideration of episodic variations of clinical pictures; this is somewhat at variance with DSM–III–R, where chronicity – even though clinically varied through acute exacerbations – is stressed).

Pronounced depressive or manic symptoms now exclude the application of this diagnostic concept, unless the schizophrenic symptoms appeared unequivocally prior to the affective ones. In the same manner more consideration is given to the schizoaffective disorders than in ICD–9 (see Chapters D3 and D4).

Finally, as in ICD–9 and all other diagnostic systems for schizophrenic illnesses, the exclusion criterion of organicity applies.

The syndromatological differentiation of the entire group takes place at the fourth position (fourth character codes). This is considerably modified in comparison with ICD–9. Disregarding the ICD–9 residual categories 295.8 (other) and 295.9 (unspecified), which, in the ICD–10 draft, correspond to F20.8 and F20.9, and disregarding rearrangements with respect to the frequency of the corresponding forms, the schizoaffective psychoses have been withdrawn from the category of schizophrenic psychoses and introduced as a separate F25 category of equal rank in the ICD–10 draft (see D4); in the same way the ICD–9 concept 295.5, latent schizophrenia, now appears as F21, schizotypal disorder (see this chapter). In exchange, F20 in the ICD–10 draft contains two syndrome concepts that ICD–9 did not recognize, namely F20.3, undifferentiated schizophrenia, and F20.4, postschizophrenic depression. Also worthy of note is that ICD–9 deals with schizophrenic psychoses (plural) whereas ICD–10 deals with schizophrenia (singular). Table 1 depicts the correspondences between the ICD–10 draft and ICD–9 and also – as an important influence in the development of ICD–10 – DSM–III and DSM–III–R.

The ICD–10 draft concept of schizophrenia is basically very similar to the one described in ICD–9, yet considerably narrower, because a one-month minimal duration of the full-blown illness is required, and because the important group of schizoaffective psychoses was withdrawn from the

Table 1

ICD-9	DSM-III/DSM-III-R	1989 draft for ICD-10
295 Schizophrenic psychoses	295 Schizophrenia	F20 Schizophrenia
.0 Simple type (F 20.6)	.1 Disorganized (295.1)	.0 Paranoid Schizophrenia (295.3)
.1 Hebephrenic type (F 20.1)	.2 Catatonic (295.2)	.1 Hebephrenic Schizophrenia (295.3)
.2 Catatonic type (F 20.2)	.3 Paranoid (295.3)	.2 Catatonic Schizophrenia (295.2)
.3 Paranoid type (F 20.0)	.9 Undifferentiated (—)	.3 Undifferentiated Schizophrenia (—)
.4 Acute schizophrenic episode (in part F 23)	.6 Residual (295.6)	.4 Post-schizophrenic depression (—)
.5 Latent schizophrenia (F 21)		.5 Residual Schizophrenia (295.6)
.6 Residual schizophrenia (F 20.5)		.6 Simple Schizophrenia (295.0)
.7 Schizoaffective type (F 25)		.8 Other Schizophrenia (295.8)
.8 Other (F 20.8)		.9 Unspecified Schizophrenia (295.9)
.9 Unspecified (F 20.9)		
		F21 Schizotypal disorder (295.5)
		F23 Acute and transient psychotic disorder (295.4)
		F25 Schizoaffective disorder (295.7)

schizophrenia group. In contrast to this, the withdrawal of the ICD–9 latent schizophrenia appears to be less significant; yet it upholds the same basic tendency, which is to restrict the concept of schizophrenia to unequivocal psychotic states (under exclusion of prodromal symptoms). These changes reflect the further development of psychopathology since the formulation of ICD–9, in the development of which the affective disturbances in 'schizophrenic' psychoses and the problematic nature of borderline symptomatology were important themes.

In 1989, the Division of Mental Health of the World Health Organization presented a draft of diagnostic research criteria for field studies. The diagnostic concepts used therein correspond naturally to those of the *Clinical descriptions and diagnostic guidelines*. The given diagnostic criteria are an attempt to formulate more rigorously the instructions in the form intended for the clinical routine. However, these diagnostic criteria correspond basically to the descriptions and instructions found in the other form.

The 1989 ICD–10 draft is superior to ICD–9 through the comprehensiveness of the descriptions of the glossary, the elaboration of diagnostic guidelines, and the possibility of a systematic classification of illness course. Its schizophrenia concept is systematically multidimensional, because information about etiology (non-organic), general symptomatology, syndromatological differentiation, and course over time is taken into account. A further important improvement is that this system shall become available in compatible versions not only for clinical use but also for the requirements of primary health care and research. Prominent scientists involved in the preparation of ICD–10 have recently referred to these various aspects (Sartorius *et al.*, 1988). The ICD–10 draft shall be presented to the World Health Assembly for approval and become officially available within the next few years. It is no longer intended to revise ICD–10 again in a ten-year cycle, but instead to carry out only small adaptations.

B7

St Louis criteria

For a diagnosis of schizophrenia, **A** through **C** are required.

A) Both of the following are necessary:

(1) A chronic illness with at least six months symptoms prior to the index evaluation without return to the premorbid level of psychosocial adjustment.

(2) Absence of a period of depressive or manic symptoms sufficient to qualify for affective disorder or probable affective disorder.

B) The patient must have at least one of the following:

(1) Delusions or hallucinations without significant perplexity or disorientation associated with them.

(2) Verbal production that makes communication difficult because of a lack of logical or understandable organization. (In the presence of muteness, the diagnostic decision must be deferred.)

(We recognize that many patients with schizophrenia have a characteristic blunted or inappropriate affect; however, when it occurs in mild form, interrater agreement is difficult to achieve. We believe that, based on presently available information, blunted affect occurs rarely or not at all in the absence of B-1 or B-2).

C) At least three of the following manifestations must be present for a diagnosis of 'definite' schizophrenia, and two for a diagnosis of 'probable' schizophrenia:

Source of criteria: Feighner, J. P., Robins, E., Guze, S. B., Woodruff, R. A., Winokur, G. and Munoz, R. (1972) Diagnostic criteria for use in psychiatric research. *Arch. Gen. Psychiat.*, **26**, 57–63.

(1) Single.
(2) Poor premorbid social adjustment or work history.
(3) Family history of schizophrenia.
(4) Absence of alcoholism or drug abuse within one year of onset of psychosis.
(5) Onset of illness prior to age 40.

COMMENTARY

In 1970, Robins and Guze described a method for achieving diagnostic validity in psychiatric illness, consisting of five phases: clinical description, laboratory studies, exclusion of other disorders, follow-up study, and family study. In a review of follow-up studies of patients given the diagnosis of schizophrenia, it was shown that poor-prognosis cases could be validly separated clinically from good-prognosis cases.

On this basis Feighner et al. (1972) established diagnostic criteria for schizophrenia. Their criteria are designed to diagnose the poor-prognosis group of schizophrenics and as such contain longitudinal features (for example, poor premorbid adjustment, insidious onset, more than six-month duration of symptoms) found to be associated with poor prognosis. They also include some cross-sectional symptoms and exclusion criteria designed to differentiate between schizophrenia and affective disorders.

The criteria were not presented as final definitions; rather, they were proposed as an initial step which should enable better comparisons between results of different research groups.

The reliability of these criteria can be further increased when a structured interview is used (Helzer et al., 1978).

The criteria consist of: psychopathological symptoms as inclusion criteria (**B1** as reported symptoms and **B2** as behavioral symptoms) and exclusion criteria (**A2**).

Non-symptomatological criteria are the following: marital status (**C1**), premorbid adjustment (**C2**), duration of symptoms (**A1**), age at onset of illness (**C5**), family history (**C3**), alcoholism or drug abuse as exclusion criteria (**C4**).

Symptoms are not scored positive if they can be explained by a known medical disease of the patient.

There are two dominant features in Feighner's criteria for schizophrenia. First (**A**), a patient needs to satisfy the duration criterion of symptoms for at least six months before the index admission. Second (**B**), delusions or hallucinations in a state of clear consciousness or disorganized thought manifested by incoherent, illogical, irrelevant, or tangential speech, blocking, loose association, or other formal thought disorder are necessary (Tsuang *et al.*, 1981).

For the third feature (**C**) only three of five are necessary. Organic and affective disorder are exclusion criteria. For a diagnosis of schizophrenia, **A** + **B** + **C** must be present.

So here, for the first time, specific diagnostic criteria constituting a very restricted concept of schizophrenia are proposed for research purposes, and, consequently, a large number of patients remain undiagnosed (here assigned to the group 'undiagnosed psychiatric illness').

Beginning with Kraepelin (1913), validation of the illness concept of schizophrenia has been sought in the course and outcome of patients so diagnosed. In several studies in which different research criteria were compared with each other, diagnostic systems containing longitudinal variables such as prior social functioning and duration of symptoms were found to be more predictive of outcome than were diagnostic symptoms based on cross-sectional symptom criteria (Stephens *et al.*, 1980). So, established chronicity predicts future chronicity (as in most other psychiatric disorders), and it remains questionable whether prognosis can be considered to be a validating criterion for a system that reserves the diagnosis of schizophrenia for patients who have already manifested established chronicity (Strauss and Carpenter, 1974; Fenton *et al.*, 1981).

Generally, in studies in which different diagnostic criteria for schizophrenia were compared with each other the Feighner criteria proved to be one of the most predictive, prognostically speaking. On the other hand, it must be taken into account that they also proved to be one of the least inclusive; this must be considered especially when performing a study with first admissions of acute schizophrenic patients (Brockington *et al.*, 1978; Endicott *et al.*, 1982; Haier, 1980; Overall and Hollister, 1979; Stephens *et al.*, 1982; Tsuang *et al.*, 1981). The Feighner criteria also serve as a basis for the 'Psychiatric diagnostic interview' (Othmer *et al.*, 1981).

B8

Research diagnostic criteria (RDC)

Schizophrenic disorder

A through C are required for the period of illness in question.

A. During an active phase of the illness (may or may not now be present) at least two of the following are required for definite and one for probable:

(1) Thought broadcasting, insertion, or withdrawal.

(2) Delusions of being controlled (or influenced), other bizarre delusions, or multiple delusions.

(3) Somantic, grandiose, religious, nihilistic, or other delusions without persecutory or jealous content lasting at least one week.

(4) Delusions of any type if accompanied by hallucinations of any type for at least one week.

(5) Auditory hallucinations in which either a voice keeps up a running commentary on the subject's behaviors or thoughts as they occur, or two or more voices converse with each other.

(6) Non-affective verbal hallucinations spoken to the subject.

(7) Hallucinations of any type throughout the day for several days or intermittently for at least one month.

(8) Definite instances of marked formal thought disorder accompanied by either blunted or inappropriate affect, delusions or hallucinations of any type, or grossly disorganized behavior.

B. Signs of the illness have lasted at least two weeks from the onset of a

Source of criteria: Spitzer, R. L., Endicott, J. and Robins, E. (1978*b*) *Research diagnostic criteria (RDC) for a selected group of functional disorders,* third edition. New York State Psychiatric Institute.

noticeable change in the subject's usual condition (current signs of the illness may not now meet criterion **A** and may be residual symptoms only, such as extreme social withdrawal, blunted or inappropriate affect, mild formal thought disorder, or unusual thoughts or perceptual experiences).

C. At no time during the *active* period (delusions, hallucinations, marked formal thought disorder, bizarre behavior, etc.) of illness being considered did the subject meet the full criteria for either probable or definite manic or depressive syndrome (criteria A and B under Major Depressive or Manic Disorders [see Chapter C6]) to such a degree that it was a *prominent* part of the illness. (See criteria for Depressive Syndrome Superimposed on Residual Schizophrenia.)

Subtypes of present period of schizophrenia

This section is for studies in which there is interest in subtypes of Schizophrenia for the present period of illness.

1a. Subtypes based on the *course* of the present period of Schizophrenia. The following four mutually exclusive categories should be considered for each subject who currently meets the criteria for Probable or Definite Schizophrenia. Note: Some subjects diagnosed initially as acute may later show a subacute, subchronic, or even chronic course.

(1) *Acute schizophrenia*: A through C are required.

    A. Sudden onset – less than three months from first signs of increasing psychopathology to any of the core symptoms (criterion **A**)

    B. Short course – continuously ill with significant signs of Schizophrenia* for less than three months

    C. Full recovery from any previous episode.

(2) *Subacute schizophrenia*:

Course is closer to that of Acute Schizophrenia than that of Chronic Schizophrenia.

Example: First episode with fairly rapid onset and duration of five months.

Example: Second episode with onset for this episode over a period of six months and full recovery from first episode.

---

* Significant signs of schizophrenia include any of the core symptoms listed in criterion **A** for schizophrenia, or other delusions or hallucinations, extreme social withdrawal, eccentric behavior, blunted or inappropriate affect, mild formal thought disorder, or unusual thoughts or perceptual experiences.

(3) *Subchronic schizophrenia*:
Course is closer to that of Chronic Schizophrenia than that of Acute Schizophrenia.

> Example: Significant signs of Schizophrenia more or less continuously present for at least the past year.
> Example: Second period following a previous period from which he did not fully recover.

(4) *Chronic schizophrenia*:
Significant signs of Schizophrenia more or less continuously present for at least the last two years.

1b. Subtypes based on the *phenomenology* of the present period of schizophrenic illness

(1) *Paranoid*:
Throughout the active period of the episode of illness the clinical picture is dominated by the relative persistence of or preoccupation with one or more of the following:

1. Persecutory delusions.
2. Grandiose delusions.
3. Delusions of jealousy.
4. Hallucinations with a persecutory or grandiose content.

(2) *Disorganized (hebephrenic)* A through C are required:

A. Marked formal thought disorder.
B. Either 1 or 2:

  1. Affect which is shallow, incongruous, or silly.
  2. Fragmentary delusions or hallucinations with content not organized into a coherent theme.

C. Not associated with marked emotional turmoil except during exacerbation.

(3) *Catatonic*:
Throughout the active period of the episode of illness the clinical picture is dominated by any of the following catatonic symptoms:
1. Catatonic stupor (marked decrease in reactivity to environment and reduction of spontaneous movements and activity).
2. Catatonic rigidity (maintains a rigid posture against efforts to move him).
3. Waxy flexibility (maintains postures into which he is placed for at least 15 seconds).
4. Catatonic excitement (apparently purposeless and stereotyped excited motor activity not influenced by external stimuli).

5. Catatonic posturing (voluntary assumption of inappropriate or bizarre posture).

(4) *Undifferentiated (or mixed)*
Period of illness meets the criteria for more than one of the previous subtypes or for none of them.

(5) *Residual*
This category should be used when an individual has had a period of illness in the past that met the criteria **A** for Schizophrenia but his clinical picture now does not contain any prominent psychotic symptoms, yet residual signs of the illness persist, such as emotional blunting, extreme social withdrawal, eccentric behavior, or mild formal thought disorder. Delusions or hallucinations may be present, but are not prominent.

If a subject who meets the criteria for Schizophrenia develops a full depressive syndrome, *without* an exacerbation of his schizophrenia symptoms, he should receive the additional diagnosis of Depressive Syndrome Superimposed on Residual Schizophrenia. If there is a flareup of the psychotic symptoms, he should receive the diagnosis of Schizo-affective Disorder Depressed Type, and the subtyping on the chronicity axis should reflect the duration of the schizophrenic-like symptoms.

A through C are required for the period of illness being considered.

A. Once had an active period of illness which met the criteria for Schizophrenia.
B. The current clinical picture does not contain any prominent psychotic symptoms, although the subject may have some delusions or hallucinations.
C. Signs of the illness have persisted (e.g., blunted or inappropriate affect, social withdrawal, eccentric behavior, strange or unusual perceptual experiences, mild formal thought disorder) since the time of the active period.

COMMENTARY

The research diagnostic criteria (RDC) were developed as part of a collaborative project on the psychobiology of depressive disorders sponsored by the Clinical Research Branch of The National Institute of Mental Health, USA (Maas *et al.*, 1980). They are described as an elaboration, expansion, and modification of the Feighner criteria (Feighner *et al.*, 1972).

The main reason a modification of the Feighner criteria for schizo-phrenia was deemed necessary is that they apparently oriented them-selves on a chronic course.

In developing the RDC, many additional diagnoses were included, such as schizoaffective disorders and a number of other diagnoses of import-ance in the differential diagnosis of affective disorders and schizophrenia. There are now 25 major diagnostic categories; many of these further subdivided into non-mutually exclusive subtypes.

Successive revisions of the RDC have been made; the latest version is dated February 1978 (Spitzer *et al.*, 1978*b*).

The RDC can be used with direct examination or with detailed case records. For further increase in reliability, a structured interview, the schedule for affective disorders and schizophrenia (SADS), has been developed (Endicott and Spitzer, 1978).

There are three versions of SADS:

1. The regular version (SADS):
   Part 1 is designed to cover a documentation of the current episode
   Part 2 is primarily for describing past psychiatric disturbance
2. The lifetime version (SADS–L):
   Similar to part 2 of the SADS except that the time period is not limited to the past and includes any current disturbance. Therefore, the SADS–L is more suitable for studies with no current episode of illness
3. Version for measuring change (SADS–C)

On the one hand the RDC for schizophrenia consist of symptomatological inclusion criteria: **A1–A7** are reported symptoms which correspond mainly to the first rank symptoms of Schneider (1959). **A8** are observed symptoms (formal thought disorder accompanied by other specific symp-toms). On the other hand, symptomatological exclusion criteria (**C**) contain the criteria (probable or definite) for a manic or depressive syndrome (criteria **A** or **B** for major depressive or manic disorders, see Chapter C6). Criterion **B** is a time criterion.

In addition to these main criteria there are subtypes based either on the course of the present period or on the phenomenology of the present period of schizophrenic illness.

For a definite diagnosis of schizophrenia the RDC require the presence of at least two out of eight specific symptoms and an illness duration of at least two weeks.

There are exclusion criteria for demarcation from schizoaffective and affective disorder. The diagnostician should consider the criteria of each of the diagnoses relevant to the study. All diagnoses are judged as 'no,' 'probable,' or 'definite.'

Since 'probable' implies more than 50% certainty, it should not be used for two mutually exclusive diagnoses for the same episode of illness (for example, schizophrenia and schizoaffective disorder, manic type). Otherwise, more than one diagnosis may be given to the same individual for the same episode of illness, or for different episodes of illness (for example, schizophrenia and alcoholism). All the conditions in the RDC (with the exception of alcoholism, drug use disorder and other psychiatric disorders) are to be diagnosed only when there is no likely known organic etiology for the symptoms.

Therefore, before the RDC can be used properly, individuals should be screened to exclude those in whom organic factors may play a significant role in the development of psychiatric disturbance. (For a more thorough description see 'Introduction and instructions to RDC,' Spitzer *et al.*, 1978*b*).

The criteria included in the RDC allow for the simultaneous assignment of subjects on the basis of episode diagnosis as well as longitudinal diagnosis, without forcing closure as to which is the most appropriate for a given patient or a given purpose.

The approach taken in the RDC schizophrenia avoids limiting the diagnosis to cases with a chronic course (unlike the Feighner criteria, an illness duration of six months is not required, see Chapter B7) but also excludes brief reactive psychoses by requiring a minimum duration of illness of at least two weeks.

B9

Diagnostic and statistical manual of mental disorders, third edition (DSM-III)

Schizophrenic disorder

A. At least one of the following during a phase of the illness:

(1) bizarre delusions (content is patently absurd and has no possible basis in fact), such as delusions of being controlled, thought broadcasting, thought insertion, or thought withdrawal

(2) somatic, grandiose, religious, nihilistic, or other delusions without persecutory or jealous content

(3) delusions with persecutory or jealous content if accompanied by hallucinations of any type

(4) auditory hallucinations in which either a voice keeps up a running commentary on the individual's behavior or thoughts, or two or more voices converse with each other

(5) auditory hallucinations on several occasions with content of more than one or two words having no apparent relation to depression or elation

(6) incoherence, marked loosening of associations, markedly illogical thinking, or marked poverty of content of speech if associated with at least one of the following:

(a) blunted, flat, or inappropriate affect

(b) delusions or hallucinations

(c) catatonic or other grossly disorganized behavior

B. Deterioration from a previous level of functioning in such areas as work, social relations, and self-care.

Source of criteria: Diagnostic and statistical manual of mental disorders, third edition (DSM-III) (1980). Washington, DC: American Psychiatric Association.

C. Duration: Continuous signs of the illness for at least six months at some time during the person's life with some signs of the illness at present. The six-month period must include an active phase during which there were symptoms from **A**, with or without a prodromal or residual phase, as defined below.

Prodromal phase: A clear deterioration in functioning before the active phase of the illness not due to a disturbance in mood or to a substance use disorder and involving at least *two* of the symptoms noted below.

Residual phase: Persistence following the active phase of the illness, of at least *two* of the symptoms noted below not due to a disturbance in mood or to a substance use disorder.

Prodromal or residual symptoms

(1) social isolation or withdrawal
(2) marked impairment in role functioning as wage-earner, student, or homemaker
(3) markedly peculiar behavior (e.g., collecting garbage, talking to self in public, hoarding food)
(4) marked impairment in personal hygiene and grooming
(5) blunted, flat, or inappropriate affect
(6) digressive, vague, overelaborate, circumstantial, or metaphorical speech
(7) odd or bizarre ideation, or magical thinking, for example, superstitiousness, clairvoyance, telepathy, 'sixth sense,' 'others can feel my feelings,' overvalued ideas, ideas of reference
(8) unusual perceptual experiences, for example, recurrent illusions, sensing the presence of a force or person not actually present

D. The full depressive or manic syndrome (criteria A and B of major depressive or manic episode [see Chapter C7]), if present, developed after any psychotic symptoms, or was brief in duration relative to the duration of the psychotic symptoms in **A**.
E. Onset of prodromal or active phase of the illness before age 45.
F. Not due to any Organic Mental Disorder or Mental Retardation.

295.x Types

The diagnosis of a particular type should be based on the predominant clinical picture that occasioned the evaluation or admission to clinical care.

295.1x Disorganized type

Diagnostic criteria

A type of Schizophrenia in which there are:

A. Frequent incoherence.
B. Absence of systematized delusions.
C. Blunted, inappropriate, or silly affect

295.2x Catatonic type

Diagnostic criteria

A type of schizophrenia dominated by any of the following:

(1) catatonic stupor (marked decrease in reactivity to environment and/or reduction of spontaneous movements and activity) or mutism
(2) catatonic negativism (an apparently motiveless resistance to all instruction or attempts to be moved)
(3) catatonic rigidity (maintenance of a rigid posture against efforts to be moved)
(4) catatonic excitement (excited motor activity, apparently purposeless and not influenced by external stimuli)
(5) catatonic posturing (voluntary assumption of inappropriate or bizarre posture)

295.3x Paranoid type

Diagnostic criteria

A type of schizophrenia dominated by any of the following:

(1) persecutory delusions
(2) grandiose delusions
(3) delusional jealousy
(4) hallucinations with persecutory or grandiose content

295.9x Undifferentiated type

Diagnostic criteria

A type of schizophrenia in which there are:

A. Prominent delusions, hallucinations, incoherence, or grossly disorganized behavior.
B. Does not meet the criteria for any of the previously listed types or meets the criteria for more than one.

295.6x Residual type

Diagnostic criteria

A type of schizophrenia in which there are:

A. A history of at least one previous episode of schizophrenia with prominent psychotic symptoms.
B. A clinical picture without any prominent psychotic symptoms that occasioned evaluation or admission to clinical care.

C. Continuing evidence of the illness, such as blunted or inappropriate affect, social withdrawal, eccentric behavior, illogical thinking, or loosening of associations.

Classification of course

The course of the illness is coded in the fifth digit:

1 – Subchronic. The time from the beginning of the illness, during which the individual began to show signs of the illness (including prodromal, active, and residual phases) more or less continuously, is less than two years but at least six months.
2 – Chronic. Same as above, but greater than two years.
3 – Subchronic with Acute Exacerbation. Reemergence of prominent psychotic symptoms in an individual with a subchronic course who has been in the residual phase of the illness.
4 – Chronic with Acute Exacerbation. Reemergence of prominent psychotic symptoms in an individual with a chronic course who has been in the residual phase of the illness.
5 – In Remission. This should be used when an individual with a history of Schizophrenia, now is free of all signs of the illness (whether or not on medication). The differentiation of Schizophrenia In Remission from no mental disorder requires consideration of the period of time since the last episode, the number of episodes, and the need for continued evaluation of prophylactic treatment.

When the course is noted as 'In Remission,' the phenomenologic type should describe the last episode of Schizophrenia, e.g., 295.25 Schizophrenia, Catatonic Type, In Remission.

When the phenomenology of the last episode is unknown, it should be noted as Undifferentiated.

Psychotic disorders not elsewhere classified

295.40 Schizophreniform disorder

Diagnostic criteria

A. Meets all of the criteria for Schizophrenia except for duration.
B. The illness (including prodromal, active, and residual phases) lasts more than two weeks but less than six months.

298.80 Brief reactive psychosis

Diagnostic criteria

A. Psychotic symptoms appear immediately following a recognizable psychosocial stressor that would evoke significant symptoms of distress in almost anyone.

B. The clinical picture involves emotional turmoil and at least one of the following psychotic symptoms:
   (1) incoherence or loosening of associations
   (2) delusions
   (3) hallucinations
   (4) behavior that is grossly disorganized or catatonic
C. The psychotic symptoms last more than a few hours but less than two weeks, and there is an eventual return to the premorbid level of functioning. (Note: The diagnosis can be made soon after the onset of the psychotic symptoms without waiting for the expected recovery. If the psychotic symptoms last more than two weeks, the diagnosis should be changed.)
D. No period of increasing psychopathology immediately preceded the psychosocial stressor.
E. Not due to any other mental disorder, such as an Organic Mental Disorder, manic episode, or Factitious Disorder with Psychological Symptoms.

COMMENTARY

The Feighner and RDC diagnostic systems are the forerunners of DSM-III (Fenton *et al.*, 1981), since their method of setting up non-ambiguous inclusion and exclusion criteria for a series of psychiatric disorders is clearly the methodological basis of DSM-III. Although it is sometimes stated that DSM-III – in contrast to the Feighner and RDC definitions – is primarily geared for more general clinical purposes than for specific research (Fox, 1981), its diagnostic criteria are no less sophisticated because they are often much more differentiated, and, indeed, much more complicated.

The decision-tree logic behind the inclusion and exclusion criteria for those clinical states traditionally considered by most to be part of the so-called endogenous psychoses is probably best exemplified by the rules of application formulated for a DSM-III diagnosis of schizophrenic disorder. This formulation requires the presence of at least one psychotic symptom from criteria A1 to A6 during an active period of illness, whereby the individual 'schizophrenic' symptom items of inclusion criteria A are more or less similar to those found in the RDC; indeed, with only one exception (item A6), all other A symptoms (A1–A5) refer solely to 'schizophrenic' delusional and hallucinatory experiences, and some of these are clearly Schneiderian first rank symptoms (Schneider, 1959).

As for item A6, it incorporates behavioral and experiential abnormalities.

In this context, it is important to note that the behavioral symptoms listed in item **A6** are more or less formulated in terms of the Bleulerian emphasis (Bleuler, 1911) on formal thought disturbance (for example, incoherence, marked loosening of associations, markedly illogical thinking), a conceptual stress also built into the RDC concept of schizophrenia. Paradoxically, however, this does not seem to make the DSM-III definition of schizophrenia 'more Bleulerian' in this respect, since item **A6** is actually very narrowly defined; as in the RDC, it can only be rated positively when found coupled with some other behavioral symptom (flat/inadequate affect (**A6a**); catatonic symptoms, disorganized behavior (**A6c**) and/or some other experience (any delusion/hallucination; **A6b**).

At first glance DSM-III's 'affective' exclusion, criterion **D**, for schizophrenic disorder seems to be quite closely related to corresponding criteria in the Feighner and RDC definitions. They are, of course, similar in that the DSM-III diagnosis cannot be made in the presence of a 'full' depressive or manic syndrome (which is fulfillment of criteria A and B for DSM-III manic or major depressive episode, see Chapter C7). However, they are different in that the relationship of any 'full' affective syndrome to the 'schizophrenic' symptoms defined in terms of the A criterion of DSM-III schizophrenic disorder is formulated much more precisely so that the **D** item of DSM-III can most likely be considered to be a less stringent exclusion criterion of 'affectivity.' This precision is because DSM-III concretely describes some additional – and more complicated – exclusion possibilities based on the intensity and chronology of the affective syndromes and symptoms entering into a coupling with the 'schizophrenic' features. For example: should a 'full' depressive or manic syndrome develop after the appearance of first rank symptoms or should it fail to dominate or persist long enough when occurring prior to psychotic phenomena then such a syndrome can no longer, according to DSM-III, serve as an 'affective' exclusion criterion. In such a clinical situation, the diagnosis of DSM-III schizophrenic disorder can still be made, whereas the Feighner and RDC systems would require dropping this diagnosis from consideration.

The chronological **C** criterion of the DSM-III definition of schizophrenic disorder is identical with that found in the Feighner concept. As in the latter diagnostic system, it also functions in DSM-III as an absolute inclusion criterion, requiring that a certain degree of illness must have persisted continuously for at least six months at some point in time. In contrast to the Feighner definition of schizophrenia, however, DSM-III clearly places weights of sorts on the 'schizophrenic' symptomatology embedded in this duration criterion. In other words: the required six-month period in DSM-III cannot be 'filled up' by prodromal and/or residual syndromes alone, but only by an active 'psychotic' segment (consisting of the presence of at least one of the 'schizophrenic' inclusion symptoms in criterion **A**) or by some combination of these prodromal, residual and active 'psychotic' syndromes. Six of the eight items, constituting the prodromal and/or residual syndromes, focus on behavior (**C1–C6**) – whereby items **C5** and **C6** are more or less the same as some of the behavioral abnormalities which form part of **A6** – whereas the remaining two items (**C7** and **C8**) represent abnormal experiences.

The authors of DSM-III maintain that their concept of schizophrenic disorder is not chiefly couched in terms of chronicity. Although it is true that the **C** criterion requiring a continuous period of illness for at least six months can be regarded as one reflecting an insidious onset and not necessarily as one denoting chronicity, the additional requirement of deterioration from a normally higher level of everyday functioning (criterion **B**) apparently favors the identification of cases with a certain tendency towards chronicity. Moreover, some of the additional terms of diagnostic classification that DSM-III uses for its subtypes of schizophrenic disorder also seem to support this interpretation. Therefore, the most important rules of application for the further subtyping of patients with DSM-III schizophrenic disorder is carried out on the basis of course features in which the primary focus is on chronicity (more than two years) and subchronicity (between six months and two years); acute exacerbations in this system, when they occur, are viewed merely as secondary phenomena of the subchronic and chronic course types. In other words, the terminology upon which DSM-III draws in defining schizophrenic disorder implies the presence of an illness that at some point in time must have been, if not chronic, at least subchronic.

As a corollary to what has just been written, there is no possibility of diagnosing an acute schizophrenic condition in DSM-III. This is also the case with Feighner schizophrenia in which the duration criterion is similar; moreover, both these diagnostic definitions contrast sharply with the corresponding rules of application found in the RDC. In the latter diagnostic system, in which the chronological inclusion criterion is one of only two weeks' duration, the diagnosis of some cases of acute endogenous psychotic illness can be accommodated within its concept of schizophrenia, namely cases in which all the criteria for a DSM-III schizophrenic disorder – with the exception of the duration criterion of at least six months of continuous illness – have been fulfilled. To deal with such situations DSM-III establishes some additional chronological criteria enabling a diagnosis still to be made, whereas in the Feighner system there are no further rules to follow should all the criteria for schizophrenia, except the chronological one, be fulfilled.

The most important of these additional chronological criteria seems to be that DSM-III classifies the patients just mentioned as having schizophreniform disorder provided that they have been ill for less than six months but more than two weeks; but should the continuous duration of illness be extended to reach the six-month limit, a re-diagnosis in terms of DSM-III schizophrenic disorder must then be considered. On the other hand, a patient with several periods of schizophreniform disorder, each terminating in recovery but *in toto* lasting for six months, is not regarded as suffering from schizophrenic disorder, since the period of illness was not a continuous one. In other words: many patients with a diagnosis of DSM-III schizophreniform disorder are most likely those who, in terms of the RDC, suffer from acute schizophrenia. Another important associated chronological consideration is that clinical states fulfilling symptomatological criteria for DSM-III schizophreniform disorder cannot be given this diagnosis when linked with a duration of less than two weeks of illness. Instead, in many similar clinical situations DSM-III also opts for diagnosing what it calls a brief reactive psychosis even when only certain 'psychotic' criteria – much less rigorous than those listed under the **A** criterion of schizophrenic disorder in DSM-III – are fulfilled in the absence of a 'full' affective syndrome; should this condition last for more than two weeks DSM-III allows a change of diagnosis into one of affective, schizophreniform, or schizophrenic disorder, depending on the clinical context.

A few cautious assumptions can be made based on what has been written so far. The concept of schizophrenic disorder in DSM-III appears to be much narrower than the corresponding RDC definition and this is probably chiefly due to the chronological inclusion **C** criterion of six months of continuous illness. Moreover, the DSM-III definition of schizophrenic disorders seems to be a bit wider than the corresponding Feighner concept (Feighner *et al.*, 1972); this most likely results from the different chronological rules of application for the full affective syndromes. In other words, the Feighner criteria, but not those of DSM-III, allow all 'full' affective syndromes to function as exclusion criteria. Indeed, the diagnostic criteria for DSM-III schizophrenic disorder or DSM-III major affective disorder (see Chapter C7) have been formulated in such a way that the diagnostician is called upon to place most cases of major functional psychotic illness on either the very wide affective or the rather narrow schizophrenic side of a dichotomy more or less reflecting a Kraepelinean diagnostic bias (Kraepelin, 1913).

B10

Diagnostic and statistical manual of mental disorders, third edition, revised (DSM–III–R)

295.xx Schizophrenia

A. Presence of characteristic psychotic symptoms in the active phase: either (1), (2), or (3) for at least one week (unless the symptoms are successfully treated):

   (1) two of the following:

      (a) delusions
      (b) prominent hallucinations (throughout the day for several days or several times a week for several weeks, each hallucinatory experience not being limited to a few brief moments)
      (c) incoherence or marked loosening of associations
      (d) catatonic behavior
      (e) flat or grossly inappropriate affect

   (2) bizarre delusions (i.e., involving a phenomenon that the person's culture would regard as totally implausible, e.g., thought broadcasting, being controlled by a dead person)

   (3) prominent hallucinations (as defined in (1b) above) of a voice with content having no apparent relation to depression or elation, or a voice keeping up a running commentary on the person's behavior or thoughts, or two or more voices conversing with each other

B. During the course of the disturbance, functioning in such areas as work, social relations, and self-care is markedly below the highest

Source of criteria: Diagnostic and statistical manual of mental disorders, third edition, revised (DSM–III–R) (1987). Washington, DC: American Psychiatric Association.

level achieved before onset of the disturbance (or, when the onset is in childhood or adolescence, failure to achieve expected level of social development).

C. Schizoaffective Disorder and Mood Disorder with Psychotic Features have been ruled out, i.e., if a Major Depressive or Manic Syndrome has ever been present during an active phase of the disturbance, the total duration of all episodes of a mood syndrome has been brief relative to the total duration of the active and residual phases of the disturbance.

D. Continuous signs of the disturbance for at least six months. The six-month period must include an active phase (of at least one week, or less if symptoms have been successfully treated) during which there were psychotic symptoms characteristic of Schizophrenia (symptoms in A), with or without a prodromal or residual phase, as defined below.

Prodromal phase: A clear deterioration in functioning before the active phase of the disturbance that is not due to a disturbance in mood or to a Psychoactive Substance Use Disorder and that involves at least two of the symptoms listed below.

Residual phase: Following the active phase of the disturbance, persistence of at least two of the symptoms noted below, these not being due to a disturbance in mood or to a Psychoactive Substance Use Disorder.

Prodromal or residual symptoms:

(1) marked social isolation or withdrawal
(2) marked impairment in role functioning as wage-earner, student, or homemaker
(3) markedly peculiar behavior (e.g., collecting garbage, talking to self in public, hoarding food)
(4) marked impairment in personal hygiene and grooming
(5) blunted or inappropriate affect
(6) digressive, vague, overelaborate, or circumstantial speech, or poverty of speech, or poverty of content of speech
(7) odd beliefs or magical thinking, influencing behavior and inconsistent with cultural norms, e.g., superstitiousness, belief in clairvoyance, telepathy, 'sixth sense,' 'others can feel my feelings,' overvalued ideas, ideas of reference
(8) unusual perceptual experiences, e.g., recurrent illusions, sensing the presence of a force or person not actually present
(9) marked lack of initiative, interests, or energy

Examples: Six months of prodromal symptoms with one week of symptoms from A; no prodromal symptoms with six months of symptoms from A; no prodromal symptoms with one week of symptoms from A and six months of residual symptoms.

E. It cannot be established that an organic factor initiated and maintained the disturbance.

F. If there is a history of Autistic Disorder, the additional diagnosis of Schizophrenia is made only if prominent delusions or hallucinations are also present.

COMMENTARY

Some important changes have been made in the original DSM–III concept of schizophrenic disorder (and its related disorders) discussed in chapter B9, and these have now been incorporated into a new DSM–III–R definition called schizophrenia.

Perhaps the most important change involves the reorganization of criterion A, the aim in general apparently being to make it simpler, and, more specifically, to take account of corresponding changes made in the DSM–III–R criteria for delusional (paranoid) disorders (see Chapters E6 and E7). The formulation of the three main symptom items of the new A criterion partially involves a shifting and partially a collapsing of the six symptom items of the original A criterion. Therefore, the original A1 (delusion) item has been retained as the new A2 (delusion) item in this process of reorganization, whereas the original A4 and A5 items dealing with hallucinations have been combined to constitute the new A3 (hallucination) item. Furthermore, the original A2 (delusion) and original A3 (hallucination) items are now more or less reflected in the corresponding new A1a (delusion) and new A1b (hallucination) items; moreover, the exclusion of certain types of delusional content as required by the original definition has also been dropped so that any type of content is now acceptable.

However, there are other aspects of this new formulation of the A1 criterion that merit even more attention. This item, which consists of five symptom parts, essentially represents a 'splitting up' of the original A5 criterion into its various components. In this new A1 item, then, the behavioral abnormalities of marked loosening of associations, markedly illogical thinking or marked poverty of content of speech are no longer defined in terms of a *sine qua non* requirement as was the case in the original A6, which means that there is no longer any mandatory coupling of these kinds of behavioral abnormality with at least one other pathological experience (delusion/hallucination) or behavior (blunted flat affect or catatonic phenomena/grossly disorganized behavior). In other words:

any combination of any of these forms of psychopathology now suffices, which is a reformulation of the original A6 that now probably globally widens the clinical boundaries of the A item.

There have also been a few essential changes with respect to the so-called 'chronicity bias' and the chronological criteria when diagnosing schizophrenic disorder (and its related disorders). For example, the new B criterion now takes into account onset in childhood, thus avoiding the term 'deterioration,' which had suggested that recovery never occurs. In addition, the requirement that the illness should begin before age 45 has also been eliminated. Furthermore, it is important to note that the new definition for schizophreniform disorder no longer states any minimal duration, and that the duration criterion for brief psychotic reaction now allows that such an episode may last as long as one month.

Another important point in the new definition of schizophrenic disorder concerns the role of the 'full' affective syndrome of the original D exclusion criterion which is now treated in the new C criterion. Although it is not easy to say precisely whether the change made here has widened or narrowed the application of the criterion involving the 'full' affective syndrome, it seems as if the new criterion may be more rigorous. For example: in the original D criterion it is stated that the manifestation of a 'full' affective syndrome during the active phase is grounds for excluding schizophrenic disorder when it is not brief in duration relative to the psychotic features; in contrast, according to the new C criterion a 'full' affective syndrome appearing during the active phase only serves as an exclusion criterion when its total duration is not brief relative to the active *and* the residual phase.

B11

New Haven schizophrenia index (NHSI)

CRITERIA

(1) a. Delusions (not specified or other than depressive)
   b. Hallucinations (auditory)
   c. Hallucinations (visual)
   d. Hallucinations (other)

(2) Crazy thinking and/or thought disorder. Any of the following:

   a. Bizarre thinking
   b. Autism or grossly unrealistic private thoughts
   c. Looseness of association, illogical thinking, over-inclusion
   d. Blocking
   e. Concreteness
   f. Derealization
   g. Depersonalization

(3) Inappropriate affect
(4) Confusion
(5) Paranoid ideation (self-referential thinking, suspiciousness)
(6) Catatonic behavior:

   a. Excitement
   b. Stupor
   c. Waxy flexibility
   d. Negativism
   e. Mutism
   f. Echolalia
   g. Stereotyped motor activity

Source of criteria: Astrachan, B. M., Harrow, M., Adler, D., Brauer, L., Schwartz, A. and Schwartz, C. (1972) A checklist for the diagnosis of schizophrenia. *Brit. J. Psychiat*, **121**, 529–39.

Scoring system:

To be considered part of the schizophrenic group, the patient must score on either Item 1 or Items 2a, 2b, 2c and must attain a total score of at least four points.

He can achieve a maximum of four points on Item 1: two for the presence of delusions, two for hallucinations.

On item 2 he can score two points for any of the symptoms a through c, one point for either or both symptoms d through e, and one point each for f and g. He can thus score a maximum of five points on Item 2.

Items 3, 4, 5, and 6 each receive one point.

Note: Where the fourth point necessary for inclusion in the sample is provided by 2d or 2e, these symptoms are not scored.

COMMENTARY

The New Haven schizophrenia index (NHSI) is an attempt to operation-alize the broad DSM–II concept of schizophrenia (Fenton *et al.*, 1981). Even if not formulated in as rigorous a fashion as the definitions, for example, of the Feighner, RDC or DSM–III criteria (see Chapters B7, B8 and B9), there is no doubt that the NHSI represents a set of 'true' modern diagnostic criteria. It is probably best suited as an initial diagnostic screening procedure, though it can also be used for conducting retro-spective studies drawing upon case files.

The NHSI is based on a rather complicated scoring system (see next three paragraphs) with four points being necessary to diagnose schizo-phrenia. Its items appear to contain only inclusion criteria. However, the paper introducing the NHSI (Astrachan *et al.*, 1972) listed the following two points of exclusion: (1) psychopathology associated with organic illness or linked to severe drug or alcoholic problems; (2) pronounced affective symptomatology. Unfortunately, there is no precise definition about which affective symptoms are meant and when the 'pronounced' threshold is reached. Moreover, in contrast to the Feighner, RDC or DSM–III definitions of schizophrenia, the NHSI does not use any chrono-logical criteria.

The NHSI regards some behavioral abnormalities (certain types of formal thought disorder, i.e., 2a, 2b, 2c) and/or certain pathological experiences (non-depressive delusions or any hallucinations i.e., 1a, 1b, 1c, 1d) as *sine qua non* or 'primary' requirements. This is similar to the rules of application for the Feighner concept of schizophrenia. In other words, these symptoms *per se* are rated positively or negatively and at least one must be present in order to make a NHSI diagnosis of schizophrenia. This is markedly different from the RDC or DSM–III systems, in which formal thought disorder must first be coupled with certain other experiences or behavioral symptoms before meriting a positive rating.

Another important feature is the fact that the 'primary' behavioral (2a, 2b, 2c) and experiential (1a, 1b, 1c, 1d) abnormalities just discussed are all given equal weights, each scoring two points when present. They are specifically weighted higher in the NHSI than all other behavioral symptoms (blocking, concreteness, inappropriate affect, confusion, catatonic behavior i.e., 2d, 2e, 3, 4, 6a–g), on the one hand, and all the remaining experiences (derealization, depersonalization, paranoid ideation i.e., 2f, 2g, 5), on the other. Each of the latter symptoms, when present, scores only one point.

It is within the group of behavioral abnormalities scoring only one point (2d, 2e, 3, 4, 6a–g), however, in which the most complicated weighting in the NHSI takes place. Namely, when the necessary fourth point to make the diagnosis of schizophrenia could be supplied by blocking (2d) and/or concreteness (2e), these none the less cannot be scored positively. In other words, when only *one* of the obligatory behavioral items (2a, 2b, 2c) or obligatory experiences (1a, 1b, 1c, 1d) are present (giving a score of 2), at least *two* of the remaining behavioral symptoms (3, 4, 6a–g) and/or experiences (2f, 2g, 5) must be elicited. Since blocking (2d) and/or concreteness (2e) are only rated positively *after* a NHSI diagnosis of schizophrenia has already been made, it seems that their inclusion among the items may really be superfluous.

This is in sharp contrast to the rules of application for diagnosing schizophrenia in the RDC and DSM–III, in which much more clinical importance is accorded to the patient's experiences. From what has been said thus far it is obvious that behavioral and experiential abnormalities are of equal clinical relevance in the NHSI, even though one group of behaviors and experiences is rated higher than another group. The result is that the 'primary' formal thought disorders (2a, 2b, 2c) in the NHSI – if the points with which they are weighted are any reflection – are on the same clinical plane as first rank symptoms, which can be rated positively in items 1a, 1b and 1d. This is certainly a strong reason for believing that the NHSI interprets schizophrenia in Bleulerian terms.

The Feighner concept of schizophrenia, like that in the NHSI, represents another diagnostic system giving certain formal thought disorders and delusions/hallucinations equal clinical weights regarding their importance for making the diagnosis of schizophrenia. However, unlike the NHSI, the remaining criteria of the Feighner definition, especially those pertaining to duration, are very strict and ensure that the above mentioned behavioral symptoms are not the crucial element in the rules of application. Therefore, when compared with the NHSI, the Feighner diagnosis of schizophrenia can clearly be viewed as one formulated more in terms of reflecting a Kraepelinian-oriented bias toward this disorder.

B12

Flexible system for the diagnosis of schizophrenia

Five (wider concept) or six (narrower concept) of the following items must be fulfilled:

(1) Restricted affect
(2) Poor insight
(3) Poor rapport
(4) Incoherent speech
(5) No waking early
(6) No depressive facies
(7) Thoughts heard aloud/thought broadcasting
(8) Widespread delusions
(9) Bizarre delusions
(10) Nihilistic delusions
(11) No elation
(12) Unreliable information

Source of criteria: Carpenter, W. T., Strauss, J. S. and Bartko, J. J. (1973*a*). Flexible system for the diagnosis of schizophrenia: Report from the WHO International Pilot Study of Schizophrenia. *Science*, **182**, 1275–8. This system is now also called the CSB–System for Carpenter, Strauss and Bartko (1973*a*).

The items used in Carpenter *et al.*'s (1973*a*) flexible system for the diagnosis of schizophrenia (CSB) were empirically derived, not primarily based on clinical intuition and wisdom, and this represents their chief strength. They were the result of statistically analyzing a large body of information elicited using the present state examination (PSE) by interviewing more than 1000 patients – in nine different countries – during the International Pilot Study of Schizophrenia (IPSS). Indeed, certain items of the CSB, not previously considered by clinicians as contributing to a reliable diagnosis of schizophrenia, were shown actually to possess this kind of quality.

Flexibility with respect to the twelve items of the CSB means that different cut-off points for diagnosing schizophrenia can be chosen arbitrarily to suit one's purposes. The fulfillment of five or six of these criteria is usually considered to be sufficient. Different degrees of certainty in identifying this disorder are reflected by the various cut-off points used. For example, the more CSB items required, the narrower the corresponding concept of schizophrenia and the smaller the number of probands positive for a diagnosis of schizophrenia in any given sample. Consequently, as the number of CSB criteria required increased from four to eight, the percentage of diagnosed schizophrenics in the IPSS fell from 90% to 23%.

The CSB makes no use of chronology, which is, in contrast, prominently built into the Feighner, RDC and DSM–III definitions of schizophrenia (see Chapters B7, B8, B9 and B10). Because of this, the CSB can probably be regarded as being less rigorous, at least in situations in which fewer items are required, than these last-named systems. Furthermore, it is important to note that none of the twelve CSB items functions as a *sine qua non* criterion for making the diagnosis of schizophrenia; this is again at variance with the rules of application for the corresponding Feighner, RDC and DSM–III concepts. Indeed, the CSB criteria are equally weighted, each able to contribute one positively rated item when absent (5, 6 and 11) or when present (the other nine).

Eleven of the twelve items of the CSB involve clinical signs and symptoms – the exception being the reliability of information criterion. Six items are related to behavior (i.e., items 1–6) and five to various experiences (i.e., items 7–11). Four of the positively formulated inclusion criteria for the CSB diagnosis of schizophrenia represent behavior (i.e., items 1–4) and four represent experiential abnormalities (i.e., items 7–10), whereas two behavioral symptoms (i.e., items 5 and 6) and only one experience (i.e., item 11) are negatively formulated.

Some critics have focused attention on the apparent irrelevancy of some of the twelve CSB items (Kendell *et al.*, 1979). For example, it is unclear why the absence of early morning awakening (item 5) or the presence of unreliable information (item 12) should merit clinical weights in this diagnostic system that are identical with that of first rank symptoms (i.e., item 7). This is in sharp contrast to the RDC or DSM–III definitions of schizophrenia where pathological experiences tend to receive much more clinical importance than do behavioral abnormalities. On the other hand, the CSB approach to giving weights is similar to that carried out for Feighner-oriented schizophrenia; yet the Feighner criteria are probably still much more stringent – at least when compared with the CSB in instances where cut-offs of four or five items are used – because of the duration criterion of six months.

The CSB has also been criticized because its cut-off point of five items for the diagnosis of schizophrenia was unable clearly to exclude the possibility of the presence of affective disorder (Kendell *et al.*, 1979). This is not surprising since the rules of application pertaining to those three items in the CSB more or less dealing with pathological affectivity were not formulated in terms of excluding a full affective syndrome as is the case for the corresponding Feighner, RDC and DSM–III definitions of schizophrenia.

B13

Present state examination (PSE)/CATEGO system

Class S+. Schizophrenic psychoses

This class contains the central schizophrenic conditions. The characteristic symptoms are:

(i) thought intrusion, broadcast or withdrawal,
(ii) delusions of control,
(iii) voices discussing patient in third person or commenting on thoughts or actions,
(iv) other auditory hallucinations (not affectively based),
(v) other delusions

If any of the first three symptoms is present, the patient is automatically allocated to class S+; similarly if *both* symptons (iv) and (v) are present. Schizoaffective subclasses can be distinguished.

Class O+. Other Psychoses

The chief symptoms are:

(i) catatonic symptoms
(ii) behavior indicates hallucinations.

Source of criteria: Wing, J. K., Cooper, J. E. and Sartorius, N. (1974) *Measurement and classification of psychiatric symptoms.* Cambridge: Cambridge University Press. This corresponds to the ninth edition of the present state examination. The tenth edition is currently under way. It will be included in SCAN (schedules for clinical assessment in neuropsychiatry). See Wing *et al.* (1990)

Patients are allocated to this class only if there are no other psychotic symptoms. This class is mainly represented in two diagnostic subgroups, simple schizophrenia (ICD 295.0) and catatonic schizophrenia (ICD 295.2).

COMMENTARY

CATEGO is a computer program for allocating psychiatric patients with functional disorders to one of several 'clinical classes' which are intended for use in research and investigations of clinical diagnosis. The classes are not themselves diagnoses and are not recommended for clinical use. The program uses psychopathological information collected by means of the present state examination (PSE), a semi-standardized psychiatric interview, and other schedules. Once the information is available the computer process is automatic and therefore completely reliable; that is, the same information always allocates a patient to an identical class (Wing, 1980).

The PSE has been developed since 1962 by John Wing and a group of his fellow researchers at the Institute of Psychiatry in London. It was revised four times before the first results were published (Wing *et al*, 1967). The seventh and eighth editions of the PSE were used in the US/UK project (Cooper *et al.*, 1972), in which American and British diagnostic habits were compared, and in the international pilot study of schizophrenia (IPSS: WHO, 1973), for which purpose it was translated into several languages. In 1974 the ninth edition, which is still in current use, was published (Wing *et al.*, 1974). This publication contains the PSE interview schedule with a glossary of symptom definitions, extra schedules such as the syndrome check list (SCL) for rating previous episodes, the aetiology schedule (AS), as a description of the CATEGO computer program. A supplementary manual was published later (Wing and Sturt, 1978) to describe a few modifications and to introduce a new technique, the index of definition (ID), for determining the threshold for defining a 'case,' particularly in population surveys (Wing *et al.*, 1978).

The CATEGO program can be used with the seventh, eighth, or ninth edition of the PSE. It consists of ten stages.

The first eight stages reduce the PSE items to 38 syndromes and eventually to six 'descriptive categories' which are not mutually exclusive. In stage nine, a decision to arrive at only one or two classes is forced; a 50-part and a 9-part classification are provided. In stage ten, history or aetiology data (which are gathered separately by using the syndrome check list and the aetiology schedule) can be included in order to arrive at a final classification which, under strictly limited conditions, can be regarded as a provisional 'diagnostic' class. The computer printout provides a tentative ICD-8 diagnosis (see Chapter B5) for use if investigators, in consideration of all the qualifications laid down in the manual, think it appropriate (for example, Bebbington *et al.*, 1981). If the final classification is based only on PSE data, this will often be inappropriate.

The basic intention of the authors of the PSE/CATEGO system was to increase the comparability of psychiatric research by offering a reliable procedure for gathering psychiatric information, and algorithms for arriving at homogeneous classes of patients.

CATEGO classes are not, therefore, 'diagnoses' in the clinical sense, nor are the CATEGO rules intended to suggest how diagnoses should be made (Wing, 1983). When based on the PSE alone, they are cross-sectional psychopathological syndromes. Their relationship to clinical diagnosis must be established through empirical research. For example, classes S, P, and O (see below) were found to be closely related to clinicians' diagnoses of schizophrenia and paranoid psychoses in two large international studies (Cooper *et al.*, 1972; WHO, 1973).

For schizophrenia the most relevant of the CATEGO classes is class S. It is primarily defined by the commonest and most reliable of Kurt Schneider's first rank symptoms (see Chapter B3): thought intrusion, broadcast or withdrawal (i), delusions of control (ii), and voices discussing the patient in the third person or commenting on thoughts or actions (iii). All these symptoms are experiential, none is observable. They were obviously chosen by the authors because of their great reliability, as very little decision is left to the judgment of the psychiatrist once the patient has reported the occurrence of a symptom. Beside class S, classes P and O are defined. Class P is based on delusions or hallucinations, not of the first rank, without a clear basis in pathological elation or depression. Class O is composed of catatonic disorders without the discriminating symptoms of classes S or P. The 'diagnostic' problems of Class S are the same as those of the criteria of Schneider (again, see Chapter B3).

Class S overrides others in the 9-part classification, following Karl Jaspers' hierarchical principle. However, the 50-part classification provides for a wider range of possibilities, including schizoaffective disorders.

The PSE/CATEGO has been of seminal value for psychiatric research, since it represents the first attempt to provide a reliable means of deriving homogeneous classes of disorder, using computer algorithms based on reliable examination and measurement of psychopathology. Its only 'diagnostic' value is that the final 9-part classification has been found to correspond to clinical practice in certain empirical studies (Scharfetter *et al.*, 1976; Wing *et al.*, 1974; Wing *et al.*, 1977). It could, therefore, be used to compare local diagnoses with those of clinicians taking part in the studies specified, if due allowance were made for sampling differences.

B14

Vienna research criteria (endogenomorphic-schizophrenic axial syndrome, Berner)

Definitive: A and/or B Present
Probable: Only C Present

A. *Incoherence*

without marked pressure or retardation of thinking or marked autonomous anxiety
   At least one of the following symptoms is required:

1. Blocking

Sudden cessation in the train of thought; after a gap the previous thought may (a) or may not (b) be taken up again

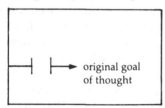
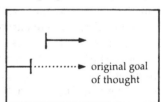

2. Derailment

Gradual (a) or sudden (b) deviation from the train of thought without gap

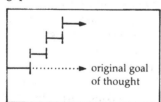
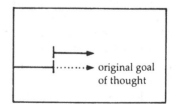

78

3. Pathologically 'muddled speech'

Fluent speech, for the most part syntactically correct, but the elements of different thoughts (which, for the patient, may belong to a common idea) get muddled together

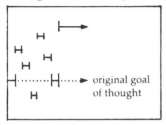

B. *Cryptic neologisms*

(inasmuch as they are not sensibly explained by the patient)

C. *Affective blunting*

(without evidence of marked depression, tiredness, or drug effect)
   This term includes flatness of affect, emotional indifference, and apathy. Essentially, the symptom involves a diminution of emotional response.

COMMENTARY

The Vienna research criteria were developed on the basis of the results of a follow-up study on paranoiac patients (Berner, 1965), which demonstrated that many of these patients were suffering from a schizophrenic or a cyclothymic* disorder. Criteria for attribution to these two diagnoses were then formulated for a further comprehensive catamnestic study on paranoiac patients constituting a part of the Lausanne Survey ('Enquête de Lausanne,' Müller, 1981). These criteria were called 'axial syndromes,' a term borrowed from Hoche (1912). The adjective 'endogenomorphic' was added to signify that the criteria in question are purely *research* ones, not to be equated to definitive diagnoses. (The formerly employed term 'endomorph' was abandoned to avoid confusion with Sheldon's (1940) physical types; 'endogenomorphic' has already been used by D. F. Klein (1974), albeit in a different sense and limited to depression).
   Two reasons were paramount for the creation of this research instrument.

* The term 'cyclothymia' is employed throughout this book as a synonym for endogenous affective disorder.

79

First of all, the diagnostic systems of the Bleulerian and Schneiderian schools (see Chapters B2 and B3), which up until then had been generally applied in German-speaking countries and whose modalities of diagnostic attribution were not clearly defined, were to be replaced, in the interests of research, by clearly and systematically definable criteria. Secondly, the Vienna criteria were to enable an investigation of the hypothesis that the diagnostic habits of both these schools attribute many cases to schizophrenia which may belong to cyclothymia or perhaps other independent illness entities lying outside the classical endogenous psychosis dichotomy. The concept of basic dynamic constellations in endogenous psychoses (Janzarik, 1959) and the research on unstable mixed states carried out by the Hamburg school (Mentzos, 1967) were especially taken into account for the formulation of the axial syndromes. The criteria were defined in 1969 and since then have undergone several modifications as a result of experience gained in their use. This book presents their current version; the endogenomorphic-cyclothymic axial syndromes will be dealt with in a later chapter.

The endogenomorphic-schizophrenic axial syndrome consists *exclusively of symptomatological criteria* primarily dealing with disturbances of expression. Formal thought disorders are *obligatory*, which means that the presence of at least one of the incoherence symptoms and/or cryptic neologisms is required. The symptoms of incoherence cannot be accurately evaluated when thought tempo is markedly accelerated or retarded or in the presence of marked autonomous anxiety; in such cases, therefore, their presence cannot be considered for diagnosis. Neologisms are to be evaluated as schizophrenic when they are cryptic; that is, possessing a purely personal meaning not sensibly explained to others. The term **affective blunting** is restricted to the sense of a global impoverishment in emotional resonance (responsiveness), and therefore, in contrast to other authors such as Taylor and Abrams (1978) and Andreasen (1979), it does not embrace parathymia (inappropriate affect). Affective blunting is difficult to evaluate in the presence of marked depression, psychic drug effects, or severe tiredness; in such cases, therefore, it should be discarded. Because affective blunting may appear as a result of these and other causes as well (unrecognized somatic illnesses, for example), which may be overlooked, its presence alone justifies only a diagnostic rating of *probable*.

The criteria are endowed with diagnostic validity not only when they are observed by the examiner but also when they are reported by the patient. The latter situation often concerns symptoms A1–A3 and C (an unequivocally reported thought arrest will be evaluated as blocking, for example). Aside from the aforementioned reserves for evaluating the criteria, no excluding criteria are employed. For gathering information necessary to confirm the presence of an axial syndrome, an expanded version of the PSE (see Chapter B13) is used.

The endogenomorphic-schizophrenic axial syndrome is a theory-oriented research instrument which is founded on the endogeny hypothesis and the schizophrenia concept of the Bleulerian school (see Chapter B2) and modifies them according to Janzarik's structural-dynamic coherency model (see Part A, Introduction). Hence the Vienna diagnostic criteria for schizophrenia are based on the following hypotheses: (1) Schneider's first rank symptoms and some of Bleuler's basic symptoms (ambivalence, depersonalization, derealization) are deemed to be expressions of dynamic instability devoid of any etiological specificity; (2) Bleuler's basic symptoms of formal thought disorder, affective blunting, and cryptic neologisms are also judged to be unspecific; however, their etiology is taken to be limited to a schizophrenic or organic origin, an assumption which is based on the experience of the Vienna research group and other authors. The question whether schizophrenia is a unique illness entity or a group of illnesses in the sense of Bleuler's 'group of schizophrenias' is left open. The Vienna school's point of view admits the possibility that various genetic predispositions and life events participate in bringing about the characteristic axial syndrome complex.

Because of these considerations, symptoms judged to be the expressions of a dynamic instability, such as first rank symptoms and some of Bleuler's basic symptoms, were excluded from the axial syndrome. Accepted for inclusion were only easily definable criteria assumed to pose the *sole* problem of demarcation from psychoses of organic origin. Consequently, despite their theoretical importance, many symptoms were left out because they could not be precisely applied. (Parathymia, for example, despite its importance in the Bleulerian dissociation theory, was left out of the axial syndrome, because in practice it could often not be distinguished from phenomenologically similar behavior seen in rapidly alternating manic-depressive mixed states). Empirically valid prognosis-indicators were dispensed with as inclusion and exclusion criteria for a number of reasons: inclusion of a time criterion, for example, was waived because this would already incorporate illness course, a criterion which could then no longer be used for the validation of the diagnostic instrument. The same arguments lead to the exclusion of genetic data. Use of indicators for good prognosis, such as confirmation of a triggering event, considered by some schools to be a sufficient reason for diagnosing psychogenic psychosis, does not appear appropriate because it is assumed that the obligatory symptoms comprising the axial syndrome do not occur in psychogenic disturbances. Besides, accepting such criteria for exclusion would contradict the possibility implicit in the working hypothesis that triggering events can call forth the illness when falling upon the fertile ground of genetic predisposition. As for the demarcation from cyclothymia, Jaspers' hierarchical principle (1963) is rejected, save the restrictions mentioned under A: the schizophrenic axial syndrome also employs no affective elements as exclusion criteria. In the occasional presence of additional symptoms pertaining to one of the endogeno-morphic-cyclothymic axial syndromes (see chapter C10), a 'schizoaffective syndrome' will be diagnosed; this judgment is purely semeiological and takes no stand as to nosological classification. Exclusion of organic or toxic causes for the symptoms is naturally a prerequisite for diagnostic application of the axial syndromes of functional psychoses.

Of all the diagnostic criteria currently employed, the Vienna criteria, by taking the concept of unstable mixed states into account, define schizo-phrenia in the narrowest terms. As the obligatory symptoms of the endogenomorphic-schizophrenic axial syndrome are often absent for considerable lengths of time during illness course, its use in cross-sectional evaluation will result in a high proportion of unclassifiable cases.

Aside from the studies mentioned at the beginning of this chapter, the Vienna research criteria were utilized in the framework of the 'Enquête de Lausanne' for the catamnestic survey of late-onset schizophrenics (Gabriel, 1977) and have been employed in studies carried out by the Vienna University Psychiatric Clinic.

B15

Taylor/Abrams criteria

CRITERIA

The criteria include all of 1–4

1) At least one of a through c

   a) formal thought disorder (driveling, tangentiality, neologisms, para-phasias, non sequiturs, private words, stock words)
   b) first rank symptoms (at least one)
   c) emotional blunting (a constricted, inappropriate, unrelated affect of decreased intensity, with indifference/unconcern for loved ones, lack of emotional responsivity, and a loss of social graces)

2) Clear consciousness
3) No diagnosable affective disorder
4) No diagnosable coarse brain disease, no past hallucinogenic or psycho-stimulant drug abuse, and no medical condition known to cause schizophrenic symptoms

Source of criteria: Taylor M. A. and Abrams R. (1978) The prevalence of schizophrenia: A reassessment using modern diagnostic criteria. *Am. J. Psychiat*, **135**:8, 945–8. Taylor, M. A., Redfield, J. and Abrams, R. (1981) Neuropsychological dysfunction in schizophrenia and affective disease. *Biol. Psychiat.*, **16**:5, 467–78.

COMMENTARY

The compilation of research criteria for functional psychoses by Taylor and Abrams (1975 *a*, *b*, 1978) emanated from an endeavor to replace the diagnostic formulations contained in DSM–II (1968) by a better-structured phenomenological approach based on exact definitions. Since the Bleulerian guidelines for diagnostic attribution (see Chapter B2) are not considered of adequate precision, Taylor and Abrams leaned mainly on the symptom descriptions by C. Schneider (1930), Fish (1967), and K. Schneider (1959), and developed their criteria out of a critical dialogue with the St Louis group.

The diagnostic criteria for schizophrenia were published in 1974 (Taylor *et al.*) and were subsequently modified to the version presented here (Taylor and Abrams, 1978; Taylor *et al.*, 1981). The criticism expressed by the Taylor group with regard to the criteria developed by the St Louis group was focused especially on differential diagnosis between schizophrenic and affective disorders and was concerned mainly with imprecise formulations. For the term 'lack of understandable speech,' they proposed a substitution of 'formal thought disorders' and they considered unfavorably the use of such criteria as 'being single' and 'poor premorbid adjustment' (Taylor and Abrams, 1975b). The correct evaluation of schizophrenic heredity was also questioned. Taylor and Abrams, on the other hand, claimed the introduction of emotional blunting as an efficaciously differentiating criterion for incorporation into the diagnostic instrument. These attempts at improvement are reflected in the above-formulated Taylor/Abrams criteria, the main purpose of which is to avoid attributing patients to the schizophrenic group when they may belong to the affective disorder group.

Except for requiring an absence of hallucinogenic or psychostimulant drug abuse, the Taylor/Abrams criteria for schizophrenia in their actual formulation contain only observed or reported criteria. Each one of the schizophrenic symptoms (1a–c), that is formal thought disorders, first rank symptoms, or emotional blunting, is considered sufficient for diagnosis. It must be kept in mind that the Taylor/Abrams criteria do not always use the same definitions for formal thought disorders as Fish (1967).

The criterion 1c (emotional blunting) encompasses two different psychopathological phenomena; namely, flattening on the one hand and parathymia (disassociated affect) on the other. In order to discredit the argument that emotional blunting has a poor interrater reliability. Abrams and Taylor (1978) developed a 'rating scale for emotional blunting.' Independently, Andreasen compiled another instrument for the same purpose in 1979. Validation of both scales provided a high interrater reliability, thereby signifying their aptitude as an ancillary diagnostic tool. It must be kept in mind, however, that both instruments use the term emotional blunting in the aforementioned application to two different phenomena.

One condition for the diagnosis of schizophrenia is clear consciousness, whereas diagnosable affective disorders, coarse brain diseases, and other somatic disturbances known to cause schizophrenic symptoms are considered to be exclusion criteria. (In his manual of 1981, Taylor required intact memory and orientation as well. Impairment of these functions is nevertheless tolerated if solely due to inattentiveness or poor concentration). The diagnosis makes use of observed as well as reported symptoms.

The Taylor/Abrams criteria for schizophrenia are largely based on pragmatic and empiric elements. The publications from this group of authors indicate, however, their attachment to the endogeny hypothesis and to Kraepelinian and Bleulerian concepts (see Chapters B1 and B2). The first rank symptoms which later replaced the items 'incomplete verbal auditory hallucinations' and 'autochthonous delusional ideas' are included in the instrument on the basis of purely pragmatical reasons. The importance attributed to first rank symptoms has none-the-less been diminished by the experience (Taylor *et al.*, 1974) that they are also observable in psychoses other than schizophrenic ones. This leads to a reversal of the hierarchical principle (see Part A) which defines the demarcation between schizophrenic and affective disorders and considers the establishment of a schizoaffective intermediary group to be superfluous. Since then, in confirmation of other publications. Taylor *et al.* (1975) also arrived at the conclusion that empirically established prognostic indicators possess poor diagnostic value; their criteria included only one of them, namely 'clear consciousness.' Genetic data have not been incorporated into the instrument because of the aforementioned reasons. The introduction of a time criterion, which Taylor and Abrams considered principally useful, was not carried through, apparently in order to preserve the illness course for validation of the instrument.

The diagnostic criteria of Taylor and Abrams are especially characterized by their exact definitions. Their concept of schizophrenia is a very narrow one. The possibility remains, as discussed in the commentary of the Vienna research criteria (see Chapter B14), that states of dynamic lability not belonging to schizophrenia might be attributed thereto, if they do not exhibit typical affective symptoms. This results from the fact that, among the psychopathological criteria, first rank symptoms may be the only determinants for diagnosis. Similarly, in cases where emotional blunting is the only psychopathological criterion present, erroneous attribution to schizophrenia may take place. In order to avoid such misclassification, Taylor and Abrams referred to Jaspers (1963) for the delimitation of reactive psychoses and to K. Schneider (1959) for demarcation from personality disorders. Neuroses, organic psychosyndromes not excluded by criterion 4, and alcoholic states should be eliminated according to the instructions of Slater and Roth (1969).

The Taylor and Abrams group have applied their criteria in various studies; those in which validation of their criteria by utilization of neuropsychological testing was attempted (Taylor *et al.*, 1975, Taylor *et al.*, 1981) should be especially stressed. Furthermore, the Taylor/Abrams criteria have been included in studies comparing different diagnostic systems.

At present the Taylor and Abrams group is working with a modified version of these criteria, which, in addition to schizophrenia, mania, and depression, include a schizoaffective entity. They have not yet been published, because further investigation will be needed to determine their usefulness.

B16

French empirical diagnostic criteria for schizophrenia

Chronic schizophrenia

A. At least two of the manifestations 1, 2, or 3 for at least two months:

   1) Major disturbance of the train of thought
      At least one of the following:

      a) loosening of associations: thought characterized by speech wherein ideas switch from one subject to another unconnected, or remotely connected, subject

      b) blocking: interruption in the flow of speech leaving the thought or an idea uncompleted

   2) Major disturbance of affect
      At least one of the following:

      a) inadequate or inappropriate affect: affect obviously at variance with the content of thought or speech

      b) affective ambivalence: simultaneous existence of contradictory affects about the same object

   3) Major impairment in reality-testing
      At least one of the following:

      a) depersonalization: impairment in perception or awareness of the self and/or derealization: impairment in perception or awareness of the outside world

      b) delusion ideas of any kind

Source of criteria: Pull, C. B., Pull, M. C. and Pichot, P. (1987*b*) Des critères empiriques français pour les psychoses. III. Algorithmes et arbre de décision. *L'Encéphale*, **XIII**. 59–66.

B. Permanent signs of the illness for at least 6 months with the constant presence of both 1 and 2:

   1) At least one of the manifestations A1, A2 or A3, or at least two of the following manifestations:

      a) vague, digressive, over-elaborate, circumstantial, or metaphoric speech

      b) marked poverty of content of speech

      c) blunted or flattened affect

      d) fantastic, illogical, bizarre, magical or delusion-toned thinking

      e) bizarre or grossly disorganized behavior

   2) At least one of the following manifestations:

      a) deterioration in level of professional, domestic, or educational functioning since the onset of the illness

      b) deterioration in social relationships since the onset of the illness

C. Onset before age 40

D. Does not meet the criteria for acute delusional psychosis

E. Not due to an organic brain disorder, alcoholism, or drug abuse

F. When an individual meets criteria A and B with the exception of the time proviso of either or both, he is diagnosed as having 'probable' chronic schizophrenia

(G.) Not due to a manic or depressive psychosis.

Acute or subacute delusional episodes considered to be schizophrenic

A. Delusional ideas of any kind

B. Acute (within the course of a week) or subacute (within the course of four weeks) onset of the delusional ideas

C. Meets the criteria A and B for chronic schizophrenia with the exception of the time proviso of either or both

D. Onset before age 40

E. Does not meet the criteria for bouffée délirante

F. Not due to an organic brain disorder, alcoholism, or drug abuse

(G.) Not due to a manic or depressive psychosis

COMMENTARY

The French empirical diagnostic criteria for schizophrenia were formulated on the basis of investigations carried out by C. B. and M. C. Pull and P. Pichot (1981, 1987*a*, *b*). The authors undertook this task to establish empirical diagnostic criteria for French nosology of functional psychoses. Until now this purpose has been definitively achieved only for the category of non-affective functional psychoses (Pull *et al.*, 1987*b*); in the realm of affective psychoses there exists to date only provisional criteria for non specific depressive syndrome (see Chapter C13). The criteria presented here concern schizophrenia exclusively; those for the remaining non-affective psychoses may be found in the section on delusional psychoses (see part E).

In order to assess the diagnostic habits of French psychiatrists concerning non-affective psychoses, 87 of them, highly qualified, were invited to select and describe several cases pertaining to this category from their records. It was suggested that they keep specific French entities in mind and that they choose only those cases whose diagnosis appeared beyond doubt. Diagnosis was not bound to any criteria in particular.

A polydiagnostic instrument embracing all specific criteria used in the realm of non-affective psychoses by important authors, past (Kraepelin, Bleuler, K. Schneider, Langfeldt) and present (Feighner, New Haven, Taylor and Abrams, International Pilot Study of Schizophrenia, Vienna research criteria, DSM-III) was developed for the survey. It is called LICET-S (Liste Integrée de Critères d'Evaluation Taxonomiques pour les psychoses non-affectives). Data gathered from 341 cases using this instrument were processed in two stages. The first aimed to single out those criteria for which a high degree of conformity emerged among the experts. These criteria served as a basis for the provisional operational definition of the French empirical diagnostic criteria for schizophrenia contained in the first edition of this book. In the second stage the provisional definitions were submitted to the clinicians who participated in the study in order to gather their criticism, comments and suggestions. The results obtained through this inquiry led to the formulation of the criteria presented here and in Chapter E1 as well as to the establishment of a decision tree for 'non-affective psychoses.'

The French empirical diagnostic criteria for schizophrenia reveal the extent to which French diagnostic habits are anchored in Kraepelinian (see Chapter B1) and Bleulerian (see Chapter B2) concepts. This becomes evident through the importance which is given to observable symptoms and evolving criteria; according to French conceptions, schizophrenia is a chronic disorder which begins early in life (at least before the age of 40) and never attains complete recovery. The characteristic symptoms included in item A may disappear in the course of the disease, but in this case at least two of the 'less typical' permanent symptoms of item B are necessary for diagnostic attribution. If the duration criteria required for the features contained in A and B are not met, the diagnosis must remain provisional. Traditional French nosology does not give exact guidelines for the differentiation between manic-depressive and schizophrenic disorders. Therefore the conception of a 'schizophrenia with thymic disorders' in the official French nomenclature (INSERM, 1968) does not imply that all disorders associating psychotic symptoms with affective ones are systematically attributed to schizophrenia. In view of this situation the item G is presented neither in an operational form nor considered obligatory and therefore has been parenthesized. Until a consensus among psychiatrists is reached in this field, it is suggested that each user of the French empirical diagnostic criteria for schizophrenia defines exactly whether or how item G is used.

The official French nomenclature INSERM distinguishes three acute delusional psychoses: the 'acute or subacute delusional episodes considered to be schizophrenic,' the reactive *bouffées délirantes*, and the true *bouffées délirantes*. The diagnostic criteria for the *bouffées délirantes* are discussed in Chapter E1. The diagnostic rules for the first of these three disorders correspond to the items A and B of the criteria for chronic schizophrenia save for the time requirement. They also limit the diagnosis to an onset before the age of 40 years. The differentation between these three states and manic-depressive disorders is handled in the same way as for the chronic schizophrenic disorders. The terms 'acute' and 'subacute' are not conceived operationally. However, authors of the system advise using the first term for episodes emerging in a time limit of not more than one week and the second for episodes appearing within four weeks. The diagnosis of an 'acute or subacute episode considered to be schizophrenic' is conceived as a provisional one, most likely to be changed to chronic schizophrenia during the course of the disorder.

The schizophrenia criteria of C. B. and M. C. Pull and P. Pichot are empirical inasmuch as they do not emanate from theoretical considerations or from purely pragmatic decisions of the authors but instead reflect the collective diagnostic experience of French psychiatrists. The studies of the authors have demonstrated that their criteria for functional psychoses have a high face- and discriminant-validity. They represent a valuable instrument to investigate hypotheses which consider the possibility of non-affective functional psychoses independent from schizophrenia.

B17

Classification of schizophrenia in the former Soviet Union (USSR)

CRITERIA

I. *Continuous schizophrenia*

  a) sluggish form (latent, pseudoneurotic, psychopath-like, paranoial);

  b) malignant juvenile (hebephrenia, malignant catatonia, malignant juvenile paranoid forms);

  c) moderately progressive (delusional and hallucinatory schizophrenia, with an onset in middle age).

II. *Periodical (recurrent) schizophrenia*

  a) with a prevalence of oneiroid-catatonic attacks

  b) with a prevalence of circular affective attacks

  c) with a mixed and changeable structure of attacks.

III. *Shift-like progressive schizophrenia*

  a) with a sluggish pseudoneurotic development and affective cyclothymic attacks;

  b) moderately progressive – with a sluggish psychopath-like development, separate paranoial disturbances in intermissions and affective delusional attacks

  c) crude-progressive juvenile forms with psychopath-like, delusional disturbances in intermissions and catatonohebephrenic attacks.

Source of criteria: Nadzharow R. A. (1967) *The clinical aspect of biological investigation of the pathogenesis of schizophrenia.* Biological research in schizophrenia, transactions of the symposium. Moscow.

In 1962, under the direction of A. W. Snezhnewski, the Institute of Psychiatry of the Academy for Medical Sciences in the USSR began research work of far-reaching conception concerning clinical and patho-genetic aspects of schizophrenia (see Snezhnewski, 1966, 1977). Partial findings were published for a Congress in Moscow by R. Nadzharow in 1967. The first summary of the results attained so far appeared in 1977.

By using the work of Kraepelin (1899 and subsequent publications) and E. Bleuler (1911), who interpreted schizophrenia as a group of related illnesses, and the general pathological concepts of hereditary diseases as a basis, one can determine the differences and similarities of pathological alterations by means of the two ideas 'nosos' (process of illness, the dynamic element of the disease itself) and 'pathos' (the pathological state, the stable alteration, the outcome of a pathological process or deficiency, the developmental deviation). In 1954, Giljarowskij suggested a concept for the classification of schizophrenic diseases, where he had already described course types. Subsequently, more weight was attributed to 'nosos'. It was hypothesized that a biological difference exists in schizo-phrenic patients, who follow these different course types (Holland and Shakhmatova-Pavlova, 1977). A. W. Snezhnewski (1977) researched further to establish the demarcation of the dynamic principles (course types), upon which the variability (unspecificity) of syndromes in the course of the main forms of schizophrenia is superimposed. As a result, more attention was devoted to following characteristics such as common features of observable development-stereotypies, age of onset, illness course, degree of evolution (proportion of productive to negative symp-toms), family history, life history and social functioning.

The characteristic, regularly progressive dynamic of the different forms of schizophrenia was described in the following way by Nadzharow (1977). The continuous type is divided into three rates of progression: malignant, moderate and mild (sluggish) course. It tends to start off in a stereotypical way with pseudoneurotic, paranoical, paranoic, paraphrenic and catatonic symptomatology. Periodic-affective symptoms or clouded consciousness must not be present at the same time. No spontaneous trend to remission. Inevitable appearance of basic negative symptoms (*Basisstörungen*), either at illness onset or after a variable amount of time.

The malignant course is characterized by an age of onset around thirteen to eighteen years. Social disability ensues within one to three years. The clinical picture is highly invariable, whatever the degree of severity the chronic progressive illness may have attained. Within this stability, the clinical picture shows a slow, relentless development over several years with the possibility of a stabilization in any stage of the course; pronounced intensity variations of the pathological features will not appear in any case.

Periodical (recurrent, acute) schizophrenia occurs mostly in women and has a good prognosis. The stereotypy in the development of the disease is from affective to delusional and to catatonic disorder. These three stages do not succeed each other, but accumulate and coexist in the deep state. There is a preponderance of mixed states and a great lability in the clinical picture with variable depth of affective symptoms. Various kinds of paranoid disorder, confusion, and dreamy states appear frequently and may coexist. This type subsumes the affective type of schizophrenia by Kasanin (1933) and the schizophreniform types by Langfeldt (1956). Obligatory signs are a good premorbid schizothymic personality with good remission after the acute phase (Sharikov, 1977).

The shift-like ('Schub') progressive form shows no connection between the severity of the attack and the character of the manifesting features. Variations of progress degree may differ in any illness stages. There is partial remission between the shifts with personality changes which are typical for this form. There also exist three rates of progression as in the continuous form. Etiological factors for the course type are postulated with endocrine insufficiency, infectious disease, family history, and psychogenic influences.

The diagnostic criteria for schizophrenia used in the USSR are purely descriptive criteria. They are the result of many empirical studies of the Institute of Psychiatry of the Academy for Medical Sciences of the USSR. The course types are not seen as definitive by the authors.

The diagnosis is attempted by application of different multiaxial modes. The individual 'axes' are the characteristic, regularly progressive dynamic (including premorbid personality), age of onset, course, degree of progress, social functioning, and etiological factors.

A paucity of narrow symptomatological criteria in course type II, and to a lesser degree in course type III, favours the hazard of overinclusion.

It is remarkable that in course type I there is no coexistence of schizophrenic and affective symptoms (exclusion criteria), but an addition of new symptoms of another hierarchy of the progress. In course type II this coexistence is allowed.

Continuous schizophrenia corresponds to Kraepelin's dementia praecox, whereas periodic schizophrenia corresponds to Kasanin's schizoaffective psychosis (see Chapters B1 and D1). Shift-like progressive schizophrenia is assumed to be a mixed form of the two.

The diagnostic criteria for schizophrenia are used in the USSR together with the ICD-9; the latter became officially accepted as diagnostic criteria in January 1983. Moreover, the glossary by Sharikov (1977) is used for cross-sectional diagnosis. The course typology is broadly applied in multidisciplinary research in the USSR.

C

AFFECTIVE
PSYCHOSES

The diagnostic criteria found in this section follow the same sequence as the section on schizophrenic psychoses. The problems posed by schizophrenia have apparently spurred the formation of theories to a greater extent than have those posed by the affective psychoses, judging from the quantity of explicit proposals devoted to each of the two themes in the literature. This discrepancy is reflected in the smaller number of systems (thirteen) for the diagnosis of affective psychoses which are presented here.

Of the classic authors in the field of psychiatry, we are presenting only Emil Kraepelin, because his immediate successors, who were included in Part B on schizophrenic psychoses, made no important contributions to the theme of this section. Next comes the International Classification of Diseases of the WHO, whose 8th and 9th revisions, in contrast to schizophrenia, are not identical, and whose April 1989 draft for the 10th revision may well be definitive with respect to functional psychoses. The three interrelated American diagnostic systems follow: first the St Louis criteria by Feighner *et al.* (1972) then, issued from them, the research diagnostic criteria by Spitzer *et al.* (1978*a*, *b*).

Both these latter systems form the basis of the diagnostic and statistical manual, third edition (DSM–III) of the American Psychiatric Association, which finds comparison with its successor, DSM–III–R. Next come the relevant categories from the PSE/CATEGO system by Wing *et al.* (1974), the Vienna research criteria by Berner and the definitions by Taylor and Abrams. The Newcastle scales make their début for reasons stated in the Introduction (see Part A). The French diagnostic criteria for non specific depressive syndrome, whose commentary also deals with the diagnostic index for specifying the type of episode, conclude this section.

Valid for all systems is that symptoms attributable to an organic illness or to the influence of toxic substances or drugs may not be included as criteria for the functional psychosis in question. Consequently, they are explicitly mentioned only when figuring as integral elements for exclusion in operational research criteria.

C1

Emil Kraepelin

I. Etiological criterion

'Whose appearance is generally unrelated to external circumstances' (Kraepelin, 1913, p. 1303),* and therefore endogenous.

II. Symptomatological criteria

Manic states

> Flight of ideas
> Heightened mood
> Increased drive

Depressive states

> Sad or anxious mood
> Thought retardation
> Decreased drive

Mixed forms

'In which signs of mania and melancholia appear simultaneously, so that pictures ensue whose traits correspond to those of both illnesses . . ., and yet they cannot be classified without ado to either one' (ibid., p. 1186).

III. Illness course

'As a rule . . . (consists of) separate attacks more or less sharply delimitable from each other or from (the normal state of) health':

---

* Quotations translated from the original German by the authors of this book.

episodic,
remitting,
and eventually relapsing,

'which may or may not resemble each other; in fact, they often represent completely antithetical pictures': monopolar, bipolar (ibid., p. 1186).

Presumably the more completely the typical symptoms and illness course present, the more certain the diagnosis will be. Yet, no formalized criterion for the decision is given.

COMMENTARY

Kraepelin's basic purpose was pointed out in the introduction to the commentary on his criteria for schizophrenia (see Chapter B1), namely 'to delineate illnesses having a common cause, symptomatology, course, and outcome' from the multitude of clinical pictures taken on by mental illnesses. Among the endogenous illnesses this endeavor concerned major affective psychoses ('manic-depressive insanity') as well as dementia praecox. In the eighth edition of his textbook *Psychiatry*, 1913, the last edition which Kraepelin wrote himself, the eleventh chapter (in the third volume: *'Clinical Psychiatry, Part Two'*) is devoted to manic-depressive insanity, endogenous dementias ('endogene Verblödungen,' known today as schizophrenia), and also to 'epileptisches Irresein' (epileptic insanity including seizure disorders). The following is drawn from Kraepelin's accomplishments presented in the eighth edition of his textbook.

Based partly on earlier German research, partly on earlier French research (see Kraepelin's general references on the subject, ibid., p. 1183), but above all on his descriptions taken from his own continually expanded comprehensive observations, Kraepelin's work united 'on the one hand the entire realm of periodic and circular insanity, on the other the simple mania, the majority of illness entities taken for "melancholia," and also a non-negligible quantity of amentia cases,' and in addition 'certain mild and mildest, partly periodic, partly chronic morbid mood modifications, which on the one hand are to be considered as preliminary stages of more severe disorders, on the other as blending into the realm of individual nature' (ibid., p. 1183) under the general concept of manic-depressive insanity.

Kraepelin phenomenologically distinguishes these last mentioned basic states ('Grundzustände,' ibid., p. 130ff) from the typical manic, melancholic/depressive, and manic-depressive mixed states (ibid., p. 1237ff). He unites them nevertheless, giving the four following reasons:

1. Experience has shown 'that despite the many external differences occurring in all the clinical pictures presented, basic traits nevertheless recur' (ibid., p. 1183). We are 'presented with a precise, limited group of disturbances . . . in all forms of manic-depressive insanity. Without being individually indicative of the illness, taken together they impress a mark of unity on the multitudinous forms taken on by the clinical pictures' (ibid., p. 1184).
2. The various illness forms merge into each other without recognizable boundaries and supersede one another in the same patient. Illnesses may resemble each other cross-sectionally; yet their courses contrast markedly (ibid., p. 1184).
3. 'A further link in common . . . is their uniform prognosis' (ibid., p. 1183). It is 'striking from general experience that the attacks of manic-depressive insanity never lead to marked dementia, . . . complete resolution of all morbid manifestations is indeed the general rule. When this is exceptionally not the case, an overall asthenia at worst develops which is as characteristic for these illness forms as it is dissimilar to dementias arising from different kinds of illnesses' (ibid., p. 1185).
4. It is pointed out lastly 'that the various forms . . . can also apparently replace one another in genetic ascendency' (ibid., p. 1185).

After exposing these reasons for combining the various illness forms, Kraepelin then presents his diagnostic criteria for manic-depressive insanity in a masterfully formulated paragraph, calling first of all on the course-typological criteria (episodic, recurrent, relapsing course; polarity of illness states), then on the symptomatological ones. Our list of criteria is taken from this paragraph.

Kraepelin's concept of manic-depressive insanity is multiaxial, drawing upon symptomatological, course (chronological demarcation of onset and termination), outcome (remission), and etiological (endogenous) criteria. The distinction between unipolar and bipolar forms is also considered; however, it is not applied systematically as a distinguishing criterion. The special weight placed on the existence of typical states and course-typological criteria is especially recognizable when characteristic states give place to the multiple variety of clinical pictures. This is mentioned once again in the conclusion under the heading 'Umgrenzung' (delimitation of the illness concept, ibid., p. 1373). Exclusion criteria follow from the Kraepelinian doctrine as a whole, above all from the notion of endogeny, and, among endogenous illnesses, from the course-typological contrast with dementia praecox (outcome difference); schizophrenic symptoms do not systematically prevail over affective ones.

Kraepelin developed his concept of manic-depressive insanity in the same way as that of dementia praecox (see his criteria for schizophrenia).

By consistently applying a general theory of illness to his observations, he succeeded in establishing a clinical psychiatric classification system which continues to be valid. Moreover, in his discussions he identified and critically examined the principal motifs which were to play a part in the ever-continuing debate over the concepts of manic-depressive illness. His concept of manic-depressive insanity, which encompasses a wide spectrum of clinical pictures, is a broad one and leaves off principally where that of dementia praecox begins. Kraepelin's concepts continue to affect all diagnostic systems.

C2

International classification of diseases (ICD), 8th revision

Psychoses (290–299)

Psychosis includes those conditions in which impairment of mental functions has developed to a degree that interferes grossly with insight, ability to meet some of the ordinary demands of life, or adequate contact with reality. It is not an exact or well-defined term. Mental retardation is excluded (310–315).

296 Affective psychoses

Includes: mental disorders, usually recurrent, in which there is a severe disturbance of mood (mostly compounded of depression and anxiety but also manifested as elation and excitement) accompanied by one or more of the following: delusions, perplexity, disturbed attitude to self, and disorder of perception and behavior; these are all in keeping with the patient's prevailing mood (as are hallucinations when they occur). There is a strong tendency towards suicide. For practical reasons, mild disorders of mood may also be included here if the symptoms match closely the descriptions given; this applies particularly to mild hypomania.

Excludes: reactive depressive psychosis (298.0); reactive excitation (298.1) ; depressive neurosis (300.4).

296.0 Involutional melancholia

Includes: an affective psychosis characterized by a severe state of depression, often with a strong paranoid component, occurring for the

Source of criteria: ICD 8th Revision (1967) WHO manual of the international statistical classification of diseases V (1965 revision). Geneva: WHO.

first time after the age of 45. The main features about bodily change (which may be bizarre); marked agitation; a sense of guilt; nihilistic delusions; delusions of poverty and impending calamity; and perceptual disturbances (especially auditory illusions and misinterpretations).

Excludes: Manic-depressive psychosis, depressed type, in which the first attack occurred before the age of 45 (296.2); reactive depressive psychosis in which the first attack occurred before the age of 45 (298.0); involutional paraphrenia (297.1); involutional psychosis NOS (299).

Inclusion terms

Involutional depression
Involutional depressive psychosis

296.1 Manic-depressive psychosis, manic type

Includes: an affective psychosis characterized by a state of elation or excitement out of keeping with the patient's circumstances and varying from enhanced liveliness (hypomania) to violent, almost uncontrollable excitement. Aggression and anger, flight of ideas, distractibility, impaired judgement, and grandiose ideas are common.

Excludes: manic-depressive psychosis, circular type (296.3), if there was a previous attack of depression.

Inclusion terms

Hypomania NOS
Hypomanic psychosis
Mania NOS
Manic psychosis
Manic-depressive psychosis:
   hypomanic
   manic
Manic-depressive reaction:
   hypomanic
   manic
Monopolar mania

296.2 Manic-depressive psychosis, depressed type

Includes: an affective psychosis in which there is reduced activity and a widespread depressed mood of gloom and wretchedness with some degree of anxiety. Close relatives are often reported to have had the same illness. There is a marked tendency to recurrence; in a few cases this may be at regular intervals. There is also an association with pyknic physique and cyclothymic temperament. Thinking and action are slowed; the patient suffers from self-reproachful and hypochondriacal delusions, shame, perceptual disturbances (especially distortion and misinterpretation of remarks overheard), and disorders of sleep, appetite, and sexual desire and capacity. Diurnal variation (symptoms worse in the morning) may be marked. Paranoid ideas are not uncommon, often taking the form of feeling shunned by others because of one's moral worthlessness. Other features may be depersonalization, perplexity, and agitation. This condition differs from depressive neurosis in the degree of severity and the nature of the delusions.

Excludes: reactive depressive psychosis (298.0); depressive neurosis (300.4); manic-depressive psychosis, circular type (296.3), if there was a previous attack of mania.

Inclusion terms

Endogenous depression
Manic-depressive reaction, depressed
Melancholia NOS
Monopolar depression
Psychotic depression

296.3 Manic-depressive psychosis, circular type

Includes: an affective psychosis that has appeared in both the depressed and the manic form, either successively or separated by an interval of normality. The manic phase is far less frequent than the depressed.
Excludes: brief compensatory or rebound mood swings in manic-depressive psychosis, depressed type (296.2).

Inclusion terms

Bipolar affective psychosis
Cyclothymia
Manic-depressive reaction, circular

296.8 Other

Includes: affective psychoses in which manic and depressive features are commingled, and other specified types of affective psychosis not classified in 296.0–296.3.

Excludes: involutional melancholia (296.0); reactive depressive psychosis (298.0); depressive neurosis (300.4).

Inclusion terms

Agitated depression
Agitated melancholia

Manic-depressive psychosis:
  mixed
  perplexed
Manic-depressive reaction:
  mixed
  perplexed

296.9 Unspecified

Inclusion terms

Affective psychosis NOS
Manic-depressive psychosis NOS
Manic-depressive reaction NOS

COMMENTARY

For general remarks concerning the ICD, see Chapter B5 on the criteria for schizophrenia presented in the 8th and 9th revisions of the ICD.

These two revisions differ in their treatment of affective psychoses. They must therefore be presented separately.

The criteria required for all forms of **psychoses** in the 8th revision apply to affective psychoses (ICD 8th revision, p. 19, see also Chapter B5). The International Glossary characterizes affective psychoses, in contrast to the schizophrenic ones, not only by their psychopathological presentation, i.e., **cross sectionally**, but also by their typical course, i.e., **longitudinally**. In referring to the latter aspect as 'usually recurrent' (ICD 8th revision, p. 32), course intermittency is only implicitly indicated, for remission of the previous episode is assumed to have occurred.

The fourth-digit code number distinguishes between only four specific forms of affective psychoses. Unfortunately, four kinds of criteria are unsystematically employed for this differentiation, namely:

296.0 Involutional melancholia
- Symptomatology: depression
- Age at onset: first occurrence after the age of 45
- Monopolarity

296.1 Manic-depressive psychosis, manic type
- Symptomatology: mania
- Monopolarity

296.2 Manic-depressive psychosis, depressed type
- Symptomatology: depression
- Age at onset: first occurrence before the age of 45
- Monopolarity

296.3 Manic-depressive psychosis, circular type
- Bipolarity
- Relapsing phases; cross-sectional symptomatology is neglected.

Polarity is the *dominating* criterion (monopolar .0 to .2, versus bipolar .3). Symptomatological types can be distinguished only within the monopolar forms (depressed type .0 and .2, versus manic type .1); a further distinction for depression is that of age at onset (first occurrence after the age of 45: involutional melancholia .0 versus first occurrence before the age of 45: depressed type .2).

Applying the ICD's general concept of psychoses, which also contains a quantitative dimension, effects the setting of two important boundaries: the first, defined in its glossary (Glossary, 1974), is that separating endogenous depression from depressive neurosis (300.4: '. . . based not only upon the degree of depression but also on the *presence* or absence of other neurotic and *psychotic characteristics* and upon the *degree* of disturbance of the patient's behavior (emphasis supplied)' (ICD 8th revision, p. 39). The second concerns the exclusion, as a criterion of bipolarity, of brief compensatory or rebound mood swings following manic or depressive psychoses. The general psychosis criterion dominates that of polarity.

The logically conceived structure of the criteria for affective psychoses in the 8th revision of the ICD comes out clearly in this integrated description. Multiaxial criteria appear here to a far greater extent than in the criteria for schizophrenia. These criteria are interrelated in a hierarchical manner, namely, criteria on an intensity axis (psychosis), a symptomatological axis of general scope (affective disturbance), and a time axis (episodic, at worst relapsing, course). In the differentiation enabled by the fourth-digit arrangement, the criterion for polarity (monopolar versus bipolar/circular) dominates symptomatological (depression versus mania) and time criteria (only for the differentiation or depressions according to age at onset). When criteria for schizophrenia coexist with those for affective psychoses, attribution to the latter illness is excluded. Such illnesses are ascribed to schizophrenia (295.7 schizoaffective type; see Chapter B5 on the ICD criteria for schizophrenia). Etiological (stress) and intensity criteria serve to exclude reactive depressive psychoses (298.0 reactive depressive psychosis, 298.1 reactive excitation) and above all, depressive neuroses (according to the criteria for this entity described under 300.4).

The concepts of affective psychoses in the 8th revision of the ICD reflect the tenets on affective psychoses prevailing when its classification system was conceived. Above all this is evident in the significance accorded to the criteria of polarity (see in particular Leonhard, 1968, also Leonhard, 1979), onset age for the differentiation of the depressive forms, and the rigid hypothesis of endogeny. Consequently, statements as to the usefulness of these criteria *vis-à-vis* their intended purpose can be made: diagnosis will comprehend only those cases whose disturbances fall into an area limited by rather narowly defined borders. Therefore, one must conclude that many probands will be excluded, although their important symptoms correspond to those of included probands.

Concerning the general evaluation of the ICD, see Chapter B5 on the ICD criteria for schizophrenia.

C3

International classification of diseases (ICD), 9th revision

Psychoses (290–299)

Psychosis includes those conditions in which impairment of mental functions has developed to a degree that interferes grossly with insight, ability to meet some of the ordinary demands of life, or adequate contact with reality. It is not an exact or well-defined term. Mental retardation is excluded (310–315).

296 Affective psychoses

Mental disorders, usually recurrent, in which there is a severe disturbance of mood (mostly compounded of depression and anxiety but also manifested as elation and excitement) which is accompanied by one or more of the following: delusions, perplexity, disturbed attitude to self, disorder of perception and behavior; these are all in keeping with the patient's prevailing mood (as are hallucinations when they occur). There is a strong tendency to suicide. For practical reasons, mild disorders of mood may also be included here if the symptoms match closely the descriptions given; this applies particularly to mild hypomania.

Excludes: reactive depressive psychosis (298.0)
reactive excitation (298.1)
neurotic depression (300.4)

Source of criteria: ICD 9th Revision (1978) *Mental disorders: glossary and guide to their classification in accordance with the ninth revision of the international classification of diseases.* Geneva: WHO.

296.0 Manic-depressive psychosis, manic type

Mental disorders characterized by states of elation or excitement out of keeping with the patient's circumstances and varying from enhanced liveliness (hypomania) to violent, almost uncontrollable excitement. Aggression and anger, flight of ideas, distractibility, impaired judgement, and grandiose ideas are common.

Hypomania NOS	Manic psychosis
Hypomanic psychosis	Manic-depressive psychosis
Mania (monopolar) NOS	or reaction:
Manic disorder	-hypomanic
	-manic

Excludes: circular type if there was a previous attack of depression (296.2)

296.1 Manic-depressive psychosis, depressed type

An affective psychosis in which there is a widespread depressed mood of gloom and wretchedness with some degree of anxiety. There is often reduced activity but there may be restlessness and agitation. There is a marked tendency to recurrence; in a few cases this may be at regular intervals.

Depressive psychosis	Manic-depressive reaction, depressed
Endogenous depression	Monopolar depression
Involutional melancholia	Psychotic depression

Excludes: circular type if previous attack was of manic type (296.3) depression NOS (311)

296.2 Manic-depressive psychosis, circular type but currently manic

An affective psychosis which has appeared in both the depressive and the manic form, either alternating or separated by an interval of normality, but in which the manic form is currently present. (The manic phase is far less frequent than the depressive.)

Bipolar disorder, now manic
Excludes: brief compensatory or rebound mood swings (296.8)

296.3 Manic-depressive psychosis, circular type but currently depressed

Circular type (see 296.2) in which the depressive form is currently present.

Bipolar disorder, now depressed
Excludes: brief compensatory or rebound mood swings (296.8)

296.4 Manic–depressive psychosis, circular type, mixed

An affective psychosis in which both manic and depressive symptoms are present at the same time.

296.5 Manic-depressive psychosis, circular type, current condition not specified

Circular type (see 296.2) in which the current condition is not specified as either manic or depressive.

296.6 Manic-depressive psychosis, other and unspecified

Use this code for cases where no other information is available, except the unspecified term, manic-depressive psychosis, or for syndromes corresponding to the descriptions of depressed (296.1) or manic (296.0) types but which for other reasons cannot be classified under 296.0–296.5.

Manic-depressive psychosis: Manic-depressive:
  -NOS   -reaction NOS
  -mixed type   -syndrome NOS

296.8 Other

Excludes: psychogenic affective psychoses (298.—)

296.9 Unspecified

Affective psychosis NOS
Melancholia NOS

COMMENTARY

Compare with Chapter C2 on criteria for affective psychoses presented in the 8th revision of the ICD.

The diagnostic criteria for affective psychoses in the 8th revision of the ICD remain unchanged in the 9th revision relative to the position they occupy *vis-à-vis* diagnostic categories other than 296, their characterization as psychoses in the ICD sense, and their general symptomatology and course typology (see ICD 9th revision, pp. 21, 29–30). In the 9th revision, though, the differentiation undertaken by the fourth-digit code number categories is more systematic. The fourth-digit code takes into account, both for manic and depressive psychoses, not only the current state (manic .0 and .2, depressed .1 and .3, mixed .4), now characterizable by the manic-depressive mixed state in addition to the two pure states, but also polarity (monopolar .0 and .1, bipolar/circular .2, .3, and .4). Therefore, the criteria of symptomatology and polarity are of *equal* consequence.

Consideration of age at illness onset for depressive psychoses has been abandoned in the 9th revision. The expressed inclusion of mild mood disorders when their symptoms correspond typologically (compensatory or rebound mood swings excluded as previously) represents a modification of the ICD general psychosis concept. Apropos, even though the introductory sentences make special reference to hypomania (ICD 9th revision, p. 30), they also call attention to depressive states. It follows logically that in its description of monopolar depression (.1), the 9th revision has abandoned the criterion quantitatively distinguishing this state from that of neurotic depression (300.4) contained in the 8th revision.

The logical structure of the diagnostic criteria for affective psychoses in general (296 without any fourth digit) is the same in both revisions. However, the fourth-digit code number criteria differ markedly. Here cross-sectional and longitudinal or course criteria (polarity) now stand side by side, equal in weight. This permits the constitution of four formally similar groups (monopolar mania, monopolar depression, bipolar mania, bipolar depression), to which a fifth one, mixed, is added, of necessity taking its place among the bipolar forms. In comparison with the 8th revision there is thus a reduction in axiality (from three to two axes, that of intensity having been abandoned). These symptomatological and course typological (time) axes are no longer related to each other in a hierarchical manner; they both have equal weight (compare with Chapter C2 on criteria for affective psychoses in the 8th revision of the ICD).

As a result of the modification brought about in the application of the ICD's general concept of psychoses to affective disorders, the diagnostic criteria of the 9th revision embrace a broader area of affective disturbances than those of the 8th. As before, however, psychoses of similar clinical presentation continue to be excluded when stress is seen to have played an important part in their emergence. The rigid hypothesis of endogeny was thus maintained. The changes reflect developments in the tenets on affective psychoses that transpired (albeit incompletely) in the intervening period. Namely, the special position occupied by 'involutional melancholia' was questioned, and less weight was given to the criterion of polarity because of variability over time (monopolar to bipolar; for example, compare the ICD 8th revision 296.2 ('depression within the limits of a manic-depressive psychosis') with the ICD 9th revision 296.1 ('endogenous depression, until now only monopolar')). Moreover, there is a greater willingness to assign mild manic and depressive mood disorders as well to the psychosis category. These criteria are therefore not only somewhat broader but also more prudent than their forerunners (compare with Chapter C2 on the criteria of the 8th revision).

C4

International classification of diseases (ICD), 1989 draft for the 10th revision

F30–F39 Mood (affective) disorders

The relationship between the etiology, symptoms, underlying bio-chemical processes, response to treatment and outcome of affective disorders are not yet sufficiently understood to allow their classification in a way which is likely to meet with universal approval. Nevertheless a classification must be attempted, and the one presented here is put forward in the hope that it will at least be acceptable, since it is the result of widespread consultation.

In these disorders, the fundamental disturbance is a change in mood or affect, usually to depression (with or without associated anxiety), or to elation. This mood change is usually accompanied by a change in the overall level of activity and most of the other symptoms are either secondary to, or easily understood in the context of, these changes in mood and activity. Most of these disorders tend to be recurrent and the onset of individual episodes is often related to stressful events or situations. This section deals with mood disorders in all age groups; those arising in childhood and adolescence should therefore be coded here.

The main criteria by which the affective disorders have been divided have been chosen for practical reasons in that they allow common clinical disorders to be easily identified; single episodes have been distinguished from bipolar and other multiple episode disorders because substantial proportions of patients have only one episode of illness, and severity is given prominence because of implications for treatment and different levels of service provision. It is acknowledged that the symptoms referred

Source of criteria: ICD–10 (1989a) *1989 Draft of Chapter V, categories F00–F99/mental and behavioral disorders. Clinical descriptions and diagnostic guidelines.* April 1989. Division of Mental Health, Geneva: WHO.

to here as 'somatic' could also have been called 'melancholic,' 'vital,' 'biological' or 'endogenomorphic,' and that the scientific status of this syndrome is in any case somewhat questionable. Nevertheless, this syndrome has been included because of a widespread international clinical interest in its survival. It is hoped that the result will be a similarly widespread critical appraisal of its usefulness. The classification is arranged so that this somatic syndrome can be recorded by those who so wish, but it can also be ignored without loss of any other information.

How to make distinctions between different grades of severity remains a problem; the three grades of mild, moderate and severe have been specified here because many clinicians wish to have them available.

The terms 'mania' and 'severe depression' are used in this classification to denote the opposite ends of the affective spectrum; 'hypomania' is used to denote an intermediate state without delusions, hallucinations or complete disruption of normal activities, that is often (but not only) seen as patients develop or recover from mania.

F30 Manic episode

Three degrees of severity are specified here, sharing the common underlying characteristics of elevated mood, and an increase in quantity and speed of physical and mental activity.

This category should be used only for a single manic episode. Previous or subsequent affective episodes, either depressive, manic, or hypomanic, should be coded under bipolar affective disorder (F31).

F30.0 Hypomania

Hypomania is a lesser degree of mania (F30.1), in that the abnormalities of mood and behaviour are too persistent and marked to be included under cyclothymia (F34.0) but are not accompanied by hallucinations or delusions. There is a persistent mild elevation of mood (for at least several days on end), increased energy and activity, and usually marked feelings of well-being and both physical and mental efficiency. Increased sociability, talkativeness, overfamiliarity, increased sexual energy and a decreased need for sleep are often present but not to the extent that they lead to severe disruption of work or result in social rejection. Irritability, conceit and boorish behaviour may take the place of the more usual euphoric sociability.

Concentration and attention may be impaired, so diminishing the ability to settle down to work or to relaxation and leisure, but this may not prevent the appearance of interests in quite new ventures and activities, or mild degrees of over-spending.

Diagnostic guidelines

Several of the features mentioned above consistent with elevated or changed mood and increased activity should be present for at least several days on end, to a degree and with a persistence greater than as described for cyclothymia (F34.0). Considerable interference with work or social activity is consistent with a diagnosis of hypomania, but if disruption of these is severe or complete, mania (F30.1 or F30.2) should be diagnosed.

Differential diagnosis. Hypomania covers the range of disorders of mood and level of activities between cyclothymia (F34.0) and mania (F30.1 and F30.2). The increased activity and restlessness, (and often weight loss) must be distinguished from the same symptoms occurring in hyper-thyroidism and anorexia nervosa; particularly in late middle-age, early states of 'agitated depression' may bear a superficial resemblance to hypomania of the irritable variety. Patients with severe obsessional rituals may be active part of the night completing their domestic cleaning rituals, but their affect will usually be the opposite of that described here.

When a short period of hypomania occurs as a prelude to or aftermath of mania (F30.1 and F30.2) it is usually not worth specifying the hypo-mania separately.

F30.1 Mania without psychotic symptoms

Mood is elevated out of keeping with the subject's circumstances and may vary from carefree joviality to almost uncontrollable excitement. Elation is accompanied by increased energy, resulting in overactivity, pressure of speech, and a decreased need for sleep. Normal social inhibitions are lost, attention cannot be sustained, and there is often marked distractability. Self-esteem is inflated, and grandiose or overoptimistic ideas are freely expressed.

Perceptual disorders may occur, such as the appreciation of colours as specially vivid (and usually beautiful), a pre-occupation with fine details of surfaces or textures, and subjective hyperacusis. The subject may embark on extravagant and impractical schemes, spend money recklessly, or become aggressive, amorous, or facetious in inappropriate circum-stances. In some manic episodes the mood is irritable and suspicious rather than elated. The first attack occurs most commonly between the ages of 15 and 30 years, but may occur at any age from late childhood to the seventh or eighth decade.

Diagnostic guidelines

The episode should last for at least one week, should be severe enough to disrupt ordinary work and social activities more or less completely, and the mood change should be accompanied by increased energy and several of the symptoms referred to above (particularly pressure of speech, decreased need for sleep, grandiosity and excessive optimism).

F30.2 Mania with psychotic symptoms

The clinical picture is that of a more severe form of F30.1. Ideas of inflated self-esteem and grandiosity may develop into delusions, and irritability and suspiciousness may develop into delusions of persecution. In severe cases, grandiose or religious delusions of identity or role may be prominent, and flight of ideas and pressure of speech may result in the subject becoming incomprehensible. Severe and sustained physical activity and excitement may result in aggression or violence, and neglect of eating, drinking and personal hygiene may result in dangerous states of dehydration and self-neglect.

In *differential diagnosis*, one of the commonest problems is differentiation from schizophrenia, particularly if the stages of development through hypomania have been missed and the subject is seen only at the height of the illness when widespread delusions, incomprehensible speech and violent excitement may obscure the basic disturbance of affect. Patients with mania who are responding to neuroleptic medication may present a similar diagnostic problem at the stage when their physical and mental activity has returned to normal levels but they still have delusions or hallucinations.

A fifth character may be used to specify mood congruency or incongruency of associated psychotic symptoms:

F30.20 Mania with mood-congruent psychotic symptoms
Hallucinations or delusions are present and are all (or predominantly) consistent with elation, such as delusions of grandiose identity, or hearing voices that carry messages of joy and power.

F30.21 Mania with mood-incongruent psychotic symptoms
Any hallucinations or delusions present are neutral to or in contrast with the elevated mood, such as delusions of persecution, reference, or control. Auditory hallucinations in the form of accusatory or threatening voices, or as a running commentary, or in the third person (as described in schizophrenia (F20)) also qualify for this code, as do other schizophrenic symptoms such as thought broadcasting and thought insertion, but if these schizophrenic symptoms are prominent and persistent, the diagnosis of schizoaffective disorder (F25) must be considered.

F30.8 Other manic episodes

F30.9 Manic episode, unspecified

F31 Bipolar affective disorder

A disorder characterized by repeated (i.e., at least two) episodes in which the subject's mood and activity levels are significantly disturbed, this disturbance consisting on some occasions of an elevation of mood and increased energy and activity (mania or hypomania), and on others of a lowering of mood and decreased energy and activity (depression). Recovery is usually characteristically complete between episodes and the incidence in the two sexes is more nearly equal than in other mood disorders. As patients who suffer only from repeated episodes of mania are comparatively rare, and resemble those who have at least occasional episodes of depression in family history, premorbid personality, age of onset, and long term prognosis, such patients are classified as bipolar.

Manic episodes usually begin abruptly and last for between two weeks and four to five months (median duration about four months). Depressions tend to last longer (median length about six months), though rarely for more than a year, except in the elderly. Episodes of both kinds often follow stressful life events or other mental trauma but the presence or absence of such stress is not essential for the diagnosis. The first episode may occur at any age from childhood to the senium. The frequency of episodes and the pattern of remissions and relapses are both very variable, though remissions tend to get shorter as time goes on and depressions to become commoner and longer lasting after middle age.

Although the original concept of 'manic depressive insanity' also included patients who suffered only from depression, the term manic depressive illness or psychosis is now used mainly as a synonym for bipolar disorder.

Includes: manic-depressive illness or psychosis.
Excludes: cyclothymia (F34.0).

F31.0 Bipolar affective disorder, current episode hypomanic

Diagnostic guidelines

(i) The current episode fulfills the criteria for hypomania (F30.0), and (ii) there has been at least one other affective episode (hypomanic, manic, depressive or mixed) in the past.

F31.1 Bipolar affective disorder, current episode manic without psychotic symptoms

Diagnostic guidelines

(i) The current episode fulfills the criteria for mania without psychotic symptoms (F30.1), and (ii) there has been at least one other affective episode (hypomanic, manic, depressive or mixed) in the past.

F31.2 Bipolar affective disorder, current episode manic with psychotic symptoms

Diagnostic guidelines

(i) The current episode fulfills the criteria for mania with psychotic symptoms (F30.2), and (ii) there has been at least one other affective episode (hypomanic, manic, depressive or mixed) in the past.

A fifth character may be used to specify whether the psychotic symptoms of the current episode are incongruent or congruent with respect to the mood:

F31.20   with mood-congruent psychotic symptoms
F31.21   with mood-incongruent psychotic symptoms

F31.3 Bipolar affective disorder, current episode moderate or mild depression

Diagnostic guidelines

(i) the current episode fulfills the criteria for a depressive episode of either mild (F32.0) or moderate (F32.1) severity, and (ii) there has been at least one well authenticated hypomanic or manic episode in the past.

A fifth character may be used to specify the presence or absence of somatic symptoms in the current episode of depression:

F31.30   moderate or mild depression without somatic symptoms
F31.31   moderate or mild depression with somatic symptoms

F31.4 Bipolar affective disorder, current episode severe depression without psychotic symptoms

Diagnostic guidelines

(i) the current episode fulfills the criteria for a severe depressive episode without psychotic symptoms (F32.2), and (ii) there has been at least one well authenticated hypomanic or manic episode in the past.

F31.5 Bipolar affective disorder, current episode severe depression with psychotic symptoms

Diagnostic guidelines

(i) the current episode fulfills the criteria for a severe depressive episode with psychotic symptoms (F32.3), and (ii) there has been at least one well authenticated hypomanic or manic episode in the past.

A fifth character may be used to specify whether the psychotic symptoms in the present episode are congruent or incongruent with respect to the mood:

F31.50   with mood-congruent psychotic symptoms
F31.51   with mood-incongruent psychotic symptoms

F31.6 Bipolar affective disorder, current episode mixed

The subject has had at least one well authenticated manic or hypomanic episode in the past and currently exhibits either a mixture or a rapid alternation of manic, hypomanic and depressive symptoms.

Diagnostic guidelines

Although the most typical form of bipolar disorder consists of alternating manic and depressive episodes separated by periods of normal mood, it is not uncommon for depressive mood to be accompanied for days or weeks on end by overactivity and pressure of speech, or a manic mood and grandiosity to be accompanied by agitation, and loss of energy and libido. Depressive symptoms and those of hypomania or mania may also alternate rapidly, from day to day or even from hour to hour. A diagnosis of mixed affective disorder should be made only if the two sets of symptoms are both prominent for the greater part of the current episode of illness, and if that episode has lasted for at least two weeks.

F31.7 Bipolar affective disorder, currently in remission

The subject has had at least one well authenticated manic or hypomanic episode in the past and in addition at least one other affective episode of hypomanic, manic or depressive type, but is not currently suffering from any significant mood disturbance. The subject may, however, be receiving treatment to reduce the risk of future episode.

F31.8 Other bipolar affective disorders

Includes: Bipolar II disorder.

F31.9 Bipolar affective disorder, unspecified

F32 Depressive episode

In typical episodes of all three of the mild (F32.0), moderate (F32.1) or severe (F32.2 and .3) forms described below, the subject suffers from lowering of mood, reduction of energy and decrease in activity. Capacity for enjoyment, interest, and concentration are impaired, and marked tiredness after even minimum effort is common. Sleep is usually disturbed, and appetite diminished. Self-esteem and self-confidence are almost always reduced, and even in the mild form some ideas of guilt or worthlessness are often present; the future seems bleak and suicidal thoughts and acts are common. The lowered mood varies little from day to day, is unresponsive to circumstances and may show a characteristic diurnal variation as the day goes on. As with manic episodes, the clinical presentation shows marked individual variations and atypical presentations are particularly common in adolescence. In some cases, anxiety, distress and motor agitation may be more prominent at times than the depression, and the mood change may also be masked by added features such as irritability, excessive consumption of alcohol, histrionic behaviour, exacerbation of pre-existing phobic or obsessional symptoms, or by hypochondriacal pre-occupations. For depressive episodes of all three grades of severity a duration of at least two weeks is usually required, but shorter periods may be reasonable if symptoms are unusually severe and of rapid onset.

Some of the above symptoms may be marked, and develop characteristic features that are widely regarded as having special clinical significance. The most typical examples of these 'somatic' (see introduction, page 84 [ICD–10, 1989 draft]) symptoms are:

(i) loss of interest or loss of pleasure in activities which are normally pleasant;

(ii) lack of reactivity to normally pleasurable surroundings and events;

(iii) waking in the morning two hours or more before the usual time;

(iv) depression worse in the morning;

(v) objective evidence of definite psychomotor retardation or agitation (remarked on or reported by other persons);

(vi) marked loss of appetite;

(vii) weight loss (often defined as 5% or more of body weight in the last month);

(viii) and marked loss of libido.

This somatic syndrome is not usually regarded as present unless about four of the above are definitely present.

The categories of mild (F32.0), moderate (F32.1) and severe (F32.2 and .3) depressive episodes described in more detail below should only be used for a single (first) depressive episode. Further depressive episodes should be classified under one of the sub-divisions of recurrent depressive disorder (F33).

Acts of self-harm, most commonly self-poisoning by prescribed medication, that are associated with mood (affective) disorders, should be recorded by means of an additional code from chapter XX External Causes of Morbidity and Mortality, Section X [see ICD–10, 1989 draft]. These codes do not involve judgements about the differentiation between attempted suicide and 'parasuicide', both being included in the general category of self-harm.

Differentiation between the mild, moderate, and severe degrees recommended here rests upon a complicated clinical judgement that involves the number, type and severity of symptoms present. The degree of ordinary social and work activities is often a useful general guide to the likely degree of severity of the episode, but individual, social, and cultural influences that disrupt a smooth relationship between severity of symptoms and social performance are sufficiently common and powerful to make it unwise to include social performance amongst the essential criteria of severity.

The presence of dementia (F00–F03) or mental retardation (F7) does not rule out the diagnosis of a treatable depressive episode, but communication difficulties are likely to make it necessary to rely more than usual for the diagnosis upon objectively observed somatic symptoms, such as psychomotor retardation, loss of appetite and weight, and sleep disturbance.

Includes: single episodes of depressive reaction, psychogenic depression or reactive depression (F32.0, .1 or .2).

F32.0 Depressive episode, mild severity

Diagnostic guidelines

Depressed mood, loss of interest and enjoyment, and increased fatiguability are usually regarded as the most typical symptoms of depression, and at least two of these three, plus at least two of the other symptoms listed above (for F32) should usually be present for a definite diagnosis. None of the symptoms should be present to an intense degree. The depressive episode must last for at least two weeks.

A subject with a mild depressive episode is usually distressed by the symptoms and has some difficulty in carrying on with ordinary work and social activities, but will probably not cease to function completely.

A fifth character may be used to specify the presence of the somatic syndrome:

F32.00   Depressive episode, mild severity, without somatic symptoms
         The criteria for depressive episode, mild severity are fulfilled, and there are few or none of the somatic symptoms present.
F32.01   Depressive episode, mild severity, with somatic symptoms
         The criteria for depressive episode, mild severity are fulfilled, and four or more of the somatic symptoms are also present (if only two or three are present but they are unusually severe, it may be justified to use this category).

F32.1 Depressive episode, moderate severity

Diagnostic guidelines

At least two of the three most typical symptoms noted for mild severity above (F32.0) should be present, plus at least three (and preferably four) of the other symptoms. Several symptoms are likely to be present to a marked degree but if a particularly wide variety of symptoms is present overall, this is not essential. The depressive episode must last for at least two weeks.

A subject with a moderately severe depressive episode will usually be able to continue with social, work or domestic activities only with considerable difficulty, if at all.

A fifth character may be used to specify the occurrence of somatic symptoms:

F32.10   Depressive episode, moderate severity, without somatic symptoms
   The criteria for depressive episode, moderate severity are fulfilled, and there are few or none of the somatic symptoms present.

F32.11   Depressive episode, moderate severity, with somatic symptoms
   The criteria for depressive episode, moderate severity are fulfilled, and four or more of the somatic symptoms are also present (if only two or three are present but they are unusually severe, it may be justified to use this category).

F32.2 Severe depressive episode without psychotic symptoms

In a severe depressive episode, the subject usually shows considerable distress or agitation, unless retardation is a marked feature. Loss of self-esteem or feelings of uselessness or guilt are likely to be prominent, and suicide is a distinct danger in the particularly severe cases. It is presumed here that the somatic syndrome will virtually always be present in a severe depressive episode.

Diagnostic guidelines

All three of the typical symptoms noted for mild and moderate severity should be present, plus usually three or more other symptoms, some of which should be of severe intensity. However, if important symptoms such as agitation or retardation are marked, the patient may be unwilling or unable to describe many symptoms in detail. An overall grading of severe episode may still be justified in such instances. The depressive episode should usually last at least two weeks, but if the symptoms are particularly severe and of very rapid onset it may be justified to make a diagnosis after less than two weeks.

During a severe depressive episode it is very unlikely that the subject will be able to continue with social, work or domestic activities, except to a very partial or limited extent.

Use this category only for single episodes of severe depression without psychotic symptoms; for further episodes use a sub-category of recurrent depressive disorder (F33).

Includes: agitated depression; major depressive episode; melancholia.

F32.3 Severe depressive episode with psychotic symptoms

A severe depressive episode which meets the criteria given for F32.2 above, and in which delusions, hallucinations or depressive stupor are present. The delusions usually involve ideas of sin, poverty, or imminent disasters, responsibility for which may be assumed by the subject. Auditory or olfactory hallucinations are usually of defamatory or accusatory voices or of rotting filth or decomposing flesh. Severe psychomotor retardation may progress to stupor.

Diagnostic guidelines

These are the same as for F32.2 above but in addition a fifth character should be used to specify whether the psychotic symptoms are congruent or incongruent with respect to the depressive mood:

F32.30 with mood-congruent psychotic symptoms

The hallucinations or delusions are entirely or very largely concerned with sin, guilt, poverty or similar topics.

F32.31 with mood-incongruent psychotic symptoms

The hallucinations or delusions are entirely or very largely concerned with topics that are not relevant to depression or guilt.

Differential diagnosis: depressive stupor needs to be differentiated from catatonic schizophrenia (F20.2), from dissociative stupor (F44.2), and from organic forms of stupor. Use this category only for single episodes of severe depression with psychotic symptoms; for further episodes use a sub-category of recurrent depressive disorder (F33).

Includes: single episodes of: psychotic depression, psychogenic depressive psychosis, reactive depressive psychosis.

F32.8 Other depressive episodes

Include here episodes which do not fit the description given for depressive episodes described in F32.0–F32.3, but for which the overall diagnostic impression is gained that they are depressive in nature; for instance, fluctuating mixtures of depressive symptoms (particularly the somatic variety) with non-diagnostic symptoms such as tension, worrying and distress; or mixtures of somatic depressive symptoms with persistent pain or fatigue not due to organic causes (as sometimes seen in general hospital liaison services).

Includes: atypical depression; single episodes of 'masked' depression.

F32.9 Depressive episode, unspecified

Includes: depression NOS; depressive disorder NOS.

F33 recurrent depressive disorder

A disorder characterized by repeated episodes of depression, as specified in depressive episode, mild or moderate severity (F32.0 and F32.1) or severe depressive episode (F32.2 and .3) without any history of independent episodes of mood elevation and overactivity that fulfill the criteria of mania (F30.1 and F30.2). However, the category should still be used if there is evidence of brief episodes of mild mood elevation and overactivity which fulfill the criteria of hypomania (F30.0) immediately after a depressive episode (sometimes apparently precipitated by treatment of a depression). The age of onset and the severity, duration and frequency of the episodes of depression are all very variable. In general, the first episode occurs later than in bipolar disorder with a mean age of onset in the fifth decade. Individual episodes also last between three and twelve months (median duration about six months) but recur less frequently. Although recovery is usually complete between episodes, a minority of patients may develop a persistent depression, mainly in old age (for which this category should still be used). Individual episodes of any severity are often precipitated by stressful life events and in many cultures both are twice as common in women as in men.

The risk that a patient with recurrent depression disorder will have an episode of mania never disappears completely, however many depressive episodes they have experienced. If this does occur the diagnosis should change to bipolar affective disorder.

Recurrent depressive disorder may be subdivided, as below, by specifying first the type of the current episode, and then (if sufficient information is available), the type that predominates in all the episodes.

Includes: (F33.0 or .1) recurrent episodes of: depressive reaction, psychogenic depression, reactive depression; seasonal depressive disorder. (F33.2 or .3) endogenous depression; manic-depressive psychosis, depressed type; vital depression; recurrent episodes of major depression, psychotic depression, psychogenic or reactive depressive psychosis.

F33.0 Current episode of mild severity

Diagnostic guidelines

(i) The criteria for recurrent depressive disorder (F33) are fulfilled and the current episode fulfills the criteria for depressive episode, mild severity (F32.0); (ii) at least two episodes should have lasted a minimum of two weeks and should have been separated by at least six months without significant mood disturbance; otherwise use other recurrent affective disorder (F38.1).

A fifth character may be used to specify the presence of somatic symptoms in the current episode:

F33.00 Depressive episode of mild severity without somatic symptoms (F32.00)

F33.01 Depressive episode of mild severity with somatic symptoms (F32.01)

If required, specify the predominant type of previous episodes (mild or moderate, severe, uncertain).

F33.1 Current episode of moderate severity

Diagnostic guidelines

(i) The criteria for recurrent depressive disorder (F33) are fulfilled and the current episode fulfills the criteria for depressive episode, moderate severity (F32.1); and (ii) at least two episodes should have lasted a minimum of two weeks and should have been separated by at least six months without significant mood disturbance; otherwise use other recurrent affective disorder (F38.1).

A fifth character may be used to specify the presence of somatic symptoms in the current episode:

F33.10 Current episode of moderate severity without somatic symptoms (F32.10)

F33.11 Current episode of moderate severity with somatic symptoms (F32.11)

If required, specify the predominant type of previous episodes (mild, moderate, severe, uncertain).

F33.2 Current episode severe, without psychotic symptoms

Diagnostic guidelines

(i) The criteria for recurrent depressive disorder (F33) are fulfilled and the current episode fulfills the criteria for severe depressive episode without psychotic symptoms (F32.2) and (ii) at least two episodes should have lasted a minimum of two weeks and should have been separated by at least six months without significant mood disturbances: otherwise use other recurrent affective disorder (F38.1).

If required, specify the predominant type of previous episodes (mild, moderate, severe, uncertain).

F33.3 Current episode severe with psychotic symptoms

Diagnostic guidelines

(i) The criteria for recurrent depressive disorder (F33) are fulfilled, and the current episode fulfills the criteria for depressive episode with psychotic symptoms (F32.3), and (ii) at least two episodes should have lasted a minimum of two weeks and should have been separated by at least six months without significant mood disturbance; otherwise use other recurrent affective disorder (F38.1).

A fifth character may be used to specify whether the psychotic symptoms are congruent or incongruent with respect to the mood:

F33.30   With mood-congruent psychotic symptoms
F33.31   With mood-incongruent psychotic symptoms

If required, specify the predominant type of previous episodes (mild, moderate, severe, uncertain).

F33.4 Currently in remission

Diagnostic guidelines

(i) The criteria for recurrent depressive disorder (F33) are fulfilled in the past, but the current state does not fulfill the criteria for depressive episode of any degree of severity, or for any other disorder in F3, and (ii) at least two episodes should have lasted a minimum of two weeks and should have been separated by at least six months without significant mood disturbance; otherwise use other recurrent affective disorder (F38.1).

This category can still be used if the subject is receiving treatment to reduce the risk of further episodes.

F33.8 Other recurrent depressive disorders

F33.9 Recurrent depressive disorder, unspecified

Includes: monopolar depression NOS.

COMMENTARY

For general remarks concerning the 10th revision of the international classification of diseases (ICD) in draft form see the corresponding chapter on criteria for schizophrenia (Chapter B6).

The section 'mood (affective) disorders' of the April 1989 draft for the 10th revision of the ICD contains, of course, the manic and depressive episodes that were classified as psychoses in the 8th and 9th ICD revisions. But in contrast to the chapters on affective psychoses in those earlier revisions this section of the ICD–10 draft encompasses a greater realm of disorders in a twofold manner. On the one hand, it no longer contains the etiological restriction to – expressed in short – endogenous disorders. On the other hand, it includes affective disorders which in the earlier revisions were to be found among the personality disorders and the neurotic disorders (above all cyclothymia and dysthymia, called cycloid personality disorder and neurotic depression respectively in the earlier revisions). Inasmuch as this book deals with psychoses, however, these personality and neurotic disorders, subsumed under F34 as persistent affective disorders, are yet clearly distinct from the characteristic unipolar or bipolar manic and depressive episodes, and consequently they shall receive no further comment. The commentary, therefore, shall treat only the categories F30 to F33.

As for the logical structure of the diagnostic concepts offered here, the code F3, which characterizes the entire 'mood (affective) disorders' section, becomes further differentiated in four ways. First of all, the third position (i.e., the second digit) characterizes course; in addition, it introduces the basic symptomatological criteria. Thus, we have (single) *manic* episode F30, *bipolar* affective disorder F31, (single) *depressive* episode F32, and *recurrent depressive* disorder F33. The fourth position (i.e., the third digit) is used for the differentiation of the episodes for both single and recurrent depressive. The fourth position can represent particular syndrome variations (presence or absence of psychotic symptoms); or severity (mild, moderate, severe). Bipolar courses can be represented not only with respect to the leading symptomatology of the current episode (manic, depressive, mixed) but also with respect to syndrome variations (for example, 'current episode manic without psychotic symptoms') or to degree of severity (for example, 'current episode hypomania'). The use of this fourth position is also pragmatic in that formal inequalities are accepted. Such defective systematics also apply to the use of the fifth position (i.e., fourth digit) for the further symptomatological differentiation, specifically with respect to mood congruence versus mood incongruence of psychotic phenomena and 'somatic' (that is, endogenomorphic) phenomena in depressive episodes. If an episode is severe, it is assumed that such 'somatic' traits are an integral part of the depressive syndrome. The fifth position is thus freed from 'somatic' attribution and can be used, therefore, for characterizing psychotic symptoms as mood congruent or incongruent when they occur.

All in all, there are multidimensionally determined categories that are described:

- By course
- With respect to the type of the affective syndrome
- With respect to its severity
- With respect to symptomatological variations

The glossary contains far more detailed descriptions of the disorders, designated with the concepts at hand, than was the case in the older revisions. They correspond to the general tenets on affective psychoses in their present state, also through the inclusion of milder forms. (This no longer stands in contradiction to a general psychosis concept as in the 8th and 9th revisions, because such a concept is absent from the 10th revision draft). The glossary also contains guidelines for establishing the diagnosis that refer to:

- The number of presenting symptoms from the series of given symptoms
- The intensity of the disorder (which should exceed that of cyclothymia, F34.0)
- The effects of the disorder in the (social) life of the patient
- The duration of the disorder to be diagnosed.

Manic and depressive episodes as well as mixed states can be registered. Under this last-named concept a categorial distinction is not made between mixed states in the narrower sense and unstable mixed states, which appear for the first time in an ICD revision, characterized through a rapid alternation of various states (see Chapter C10). Dysphoria (irritability) is mentioned as a symptomatological variation not only in manic but also in depressive episodes, but this mood disorder is not recognized as a separate entity (see Chapter C10).

With the categories F30 and F33 from the section 'mood (affective) disorders', F30 to F39, taken into account here, a broader spectrum of affective disorders is embraced than with the concepts for affective psychoses in the 8th and 9th ICD revisions, above all through the inclusion of milder forms and of illnesses with psychotic symptoms incongruent to the mood. (Nevertheless, these symptoms should not overshadow those of the affective disorder itself; were they to share the foreground and pertain to schizophrenia, a possibility mentioned only under mania, a schizoaffective disorder should be diagnosed, see Chapter D4). Both correspond to the current scientific state of the problem. That hypomanic swings following immediately upon depressive episodes receive no classificatory weight with respect to bipolarity also corresponds at least to a widespread opinion; the presence of such aftermath swings is rather compatible with the diagnosis of a unipolar recurrent depressive illness.

As for the draft of the diagnostic criteria for research (ICD–10, 1989b), the remarks that were made in Chapter B6 on schizophrenic psychoses apply here also.

C5

St Louis criteria

Primary depression

For a diagnosis of depression, **A** through **C** are required.

A) Dysphoric mood characterized by symptoms such as the following: depressed, sad, blue, despondent, hopeless, 'down in the dumps,' irritable, fearful, worried, or discouraged.

B) At least five of the following criteria are required for 'definite' depression; four are required for 'probable' depression.

   (1) Poor appetite or weight loss (positive if 2 lb a week or 10 lb or more a year when not dieting).
   (2) Sleep difficulty (include insomnia or hypersomnia).
   (3) Loss of energy, e.g., fatigability, tiredness.
   (4) Agitation or retardation.
   (5) Loss of interest in usual activities, or decrease in sexual drive.
   (6) Feelings of self-reproach or guilt (either may be delusional).
   (7) Complaints of or actual diminished ability to think or concentrate, such as slow thinking or mixed-up thoughts.
   (8) Recurrent thoughts of death or suicide, including thoughts of wishing to be dead.

C) A psychiatric illness lasting at least one month with no preexisting psychiatric conditions such as schizophrenia, anxiety neuroses, phobia, neurosis, obsessive-compulsive neurosis, hysteria, alcoholism, drug dependency, antisocial personality, homosexuality and other sexual deviations, mental retardation, or organic brain syn-

Source of criteria: Feighner, J. P., Robins, E., Guze, S. B., Woodruff, R. A., Winokur, G. and Munoz, R. (1972) Diagnostic criteria for use in psychiatric research. Arch. Gen. Psychiat., **26**, 57–63.

drome (Patients with life-threatening or incapacitating medical illness preceding and paralleling the depression do not receive the diagnosis of primary depression.) There are patients who fulfill the above criteria, but also have a massive or peculiar alteration of perception and thinking as a major manifestation of their illness. These patients are classified as having an 'undiagnosed psychiatric disorder' and are included in neither 'primary affective disorder' nor 'schizophrenia.'

In 1979 and 1981 Feighner described an additional criterion **D** which replaces the last two sentences by the following:

D) There are patients who fulfill the above criteria, but who also have a massive or peculiar alteration of perception and thinking as a major manifestation of their illness. These patients are currently classified as having a schizoaffective psychosis (Feighner, 1979, 1981).

Secondary depression

Secondary depression, 'definite' or 'probable,' is defined in the same way as primary depression, except that it occurs with one of the following:

(1) A preexisting non-affective psychiatric illness which may or may not still be present.
(2) A life-threatening or incapacitating medical illness which precedes and parallels the symptoms of depression.

The St. Louis Group now no longer makes a diagnosis of secondary depression because of a preexisting life-threatening condition (Spitzer *et al.*, 1978*b*).

Mania

For a diagnosis of mania, **A** through **C** are required.

A) Euphoria or irritability.
B) At least three of the following symptom categories must also be present.

(1) Hyperactivity (includes motor, social, and sexual activity).
(2) Push of speech (pressure to keep talking).
(3) Flight of ideas (racing thoughts).
(4) Grandiosity (may be delusional).
(5) Decreased sleep.
(6) Distractibility.

C) A psychiatric illness lasting at least two weeks with no preexisting psychiatric conditions such as schizophrenia, anxiety neurosis, phobia, neurosis, obsessive-compulsive neurosis, hysteria, alcoholism, drug dependency, antisocial personality, homosexuality and other sexual deviations, mental retardation, or organic brain syndrome.

There are patients who fulfill the above criteria, but also have a massive or peculiar alteration of perception and thinking as a major manifestation of their illness. These patients are classified as having an 'undiagnosed psychiatric disorder' and are included in neither primary affective disorder nor schizophrenia.

In 1979 and 1981 Feighner described an additional criterion **D** which replaces the last two sentences by the following:

D) There are patients who fulfill the above criteria, but who also have a massive or peculiar alteration of perception and thinking as a major manifestation of their illness. These patients are currently classified as having a schizoaffective psychosis (Feighner, 1979, 1981).

COMMENTARY

Because of the lack of meaningful and standardized diagnostic schemata suitable for current psychiatric research, Feighner *et al.* (1972) published specific operational diagnostic criteria for fourteen psychiatric disorders (see also Chapter B7 on Feighner's diagnostic criteria for schizophrenia). The introduction of the concept of 'primary' and 'secondary' affective disorder created a basis for classification which avoided etiological implications (Robins *et al.*, 1972).

Primary affective disorder is an affective illness (a mania or a depression) which occurs in an individual who has never had another kind of psychiatric illness. Depressions are described as secondary if the patient's history encompasses psychiatric disorders other than depression or mania.

The criteria for primary depression consist on the one hand of symptomatological criteria (**A**, **B**) all of which are reported symptoms, and on the other hand of a time criterion (illness lasting at least one month) and exclusion criteria (**C**) with respect to preexisting psychiatric conditions. **A** and **B** are equal in primary and secondary depression; **C** (an exclusion in primary depression) is an inclusion criterion in secondary depression. In 1979 and 1981, Feighner described an additional criterion (**D**) for differentiation from schizoaffective disorder (which in 1972 was part of the group 'undiagnosed psychiatric illness' (Feighner *et al.*, 1972)).

The criteria for mania consist on the one hand of symptomatological criteria (the authors do not specify if they are reported or observed symptoms but it can be assumed that **B**3 is an observed symptom and that **B**4 and **B**5 are reported and/or observed), and on the other hand of a non-symptomatological criterion: a time dimension in **C** (illness lasting at least two weeks). **C** also focuses on exclusion criteria and the problem of classification of patients with alteration of perception and thinking as a major manifestation of their illness.

For primary depression, a dysphoric mood and a duration of the illness of at least one month must be present; additionally at least five of eight criteria for definite depression (and four of eight for probable) are required.

So-called 'schizophrenic' symptoms were excluded from the diagnosis of depression in 1972 (Feighner *et al.*, 1972); those patients were diagnosed as having an 'undiagnosed psychiatric disorder.' In 1979, Feighner assigned those patients to the new category of schizoaffective disorder (Feighner, 1979, 1981).

For mania, euphoria or irritability and a duration of illness of at least two weeks are necessary; additionally, three of six symptom categories of **B** must be present. **C** deals with exclusion criteria. In 1972, patients with additional alteration of perception and thinking as a major manifestation of their illness were classified as having an undiagnosed psychiatric disorder (Feighner *et al.*, 1972); in 1979, these patients were assigned to the new category of schizoaffective disorder (Feighner, 1979, 1981).

In Feighner's system of classification, the differentiation between primary and secondary depressive illness is made prior to all other diagnostic decisions.

The problems of the concept of 'secondary depression' are discussed by Roth (1981) and van Praag (1982): these authors criticize this concept for its implication that alcoholism, drug dependence, anxiety neurosis, etc. are 'primary' in an etiological sense. In his critique on the criteria of 'primary' depression, Roth (1981) states that these criteria are not very specific and are bound to encompass a much wider range than the European bipolar–unipolar concept.

This is also confirmed indirectly by Winokur (1981), who reports a study showing a prevalence of 8% of primary affective disorder in a general population.

In addition, Feighner (1979) is using a further subclassification of primary affective disorders into bipolar and unipolar subtypes based upon family history and the patient's longitudinal history.

The bipolar–unipolar classification was introduced by Leonhard (1968) and validated by Angst (1966), Perris (1966), and Winokur et al. (1969), cited in Feighner (1981):

(1) Bipolar I (with mania)
(2) Bipolar II (with hypomania)

(3) Unipolar mania
(4) Unipolar depression with positive family history for mania
(5) Unipolar depression with negative family history for mania

C6

Research diagnostic criteria (RDC)

Manic disorder

(May immediately precede or follow Major Depressive Disorder.)
A through E are required for the episode of illness being considered.

A. One or more distinct periods with a predominantly elevated, expansive, or irritable mood. The elevated, expansive, or irritable mood must be a prominent part of the illness and relatively persistent although it may alternate with depressive mood. Do not include if apparently due to alcohol or drug use.

B. If mood is elevated or expansive, at least three of the following symptom categories must be definitely present to a significant degree, four if mood is only irritable. (For past episodes, because of memory difficulty, one less symptom is required.) Do not include if apparently due to alcohol or drug use.

   (1) More active than usual – either socially, at work, at home, sexually, or physically restless.
   (2) More talkative than usual or felt a pressure to keep talking.
   (3) Flight of ideas or subjective experience that thoughts are racing.
   (4) Inflated self-esteem (grandiosity, which may be delusional).
   (5) Decreased need for sleep.
   (6) Distractibility, i.e., attention is too easily drawn to unimportant or irrelevant external stimuli.
   (7) Excessive involvement in activities without recognizing the high potential for painful consequences, e.g., buying sprees, sexual indiscretions, foolish business investments, reckless driving.

Source of criteria: Spitzer, R. L., Endicott, J. and Robins, E. (1978*b*) *Research diagnostic criteria (RDC) for a selected group of functional disorders*, third edition. New York State Psychiatric Institute.

C. Overall disturbance is so severe that at least one of the following is present:

(1) Meaningful conversation is impossible.
(2) Serious impairment socially, with family, at home, at school, or at work.
(3) In the absence of (1) or (2), hospitalization.

D. Duration of manic features of at least one week beginning with the first noticeable change in the subject's usual condition (or any duration if hospitalized). If became 'mania' after hospitalization, the rater should differentiate between manic and hypomanic periods on the basis of apparent severity.

E. None of the following which suggest Schizophrenia is present. (Do not include if apparently due to alcohol or drug use.)

(1) Delusions of being controlled (or influenced), or thought broadcasting, insertion, or withdrawal.
(2) Non-affective hallucinations of any type throughout the day for several days or intermittently throughout a one week period.
(3) Auditory hallucinations in which either a voice keeps up a running commentary on the subject's behaviors or thoughts as they occur, or two or more voices converse with each other.
(4) At some time during the period of illness had more than one week when he exhibited no prominent depressive or manic symptoms but had delusions or hallucinations.
(5) At some time during the period of illness had more than one week when he exhibited no prominent manic symptoms but had several instances of marked formal thought disorder, accompanied by either blunted or inappropriate affect, delusions or hallucinations of any type, or grossly disorganized behavior.

Hypomanic disorder

(May immediately precede or follow Major Depressive Disorder.)
A through D are required.

A. Has had a distinct period with predominantly elevated, expansive, or irritable mood. The elevated, expansive, or irritable mood must be relatively persistent or occur frequently. It may alternate with depressive mood. Do not include if mood change is apparently due to alcohol or drug use.

B. If the mood is elevated or expansive, at least two of the symptoms noted in Manic Disorder **B** must be present, three symptoms if mood is only irritable.

C. Duration of mood disturbance at least two days. Definite if elevated, expansive, or irritable mood lasted for one week, probable if two to six days.

D. The episode being considered does not meet the criteria for Schizophrenia, Schizo-affective Disorder, or Manic Disorder.

Bipolar depression with mania (bipolar 1)

At some time in his life has met the criteria for Manic Disorder and Major Depressive Disorder, Minor Depressive Disorder, or Intermittent Depressive Disorder. Probable if the Manic Disorder is only probable.

Bipolar depression with hypomania (bipolar 2)

At some time in his life has met the criteria for both Hypomanic and Major Depressive Disorder, Minor Depressive Disorder, or Intermittent Depressive Disorder, and has never met the criteria for Manic Disorder. Probable if the Hypomanic Disorder is only probable.

Major depressive disorder

(May immediately precede or follow Manic Disorder.)
A through F are required for the episode of illness being considered.

A. One or more distinct periods with dysphoric mood or pervasive loss of interest or pleasure. The disturbance is characterized by symptoms such as the following: depressed, sad, blue, hopeless, low, down in the dumps, 'don't care anymore,' or irritable. The disturbance must be prominent and relatively persistent but not necessarily the most dominant symptom. It does not include momentary shifts from one dysphoric mood to another dysphoric mood, e.g., anxiety to depression to anger, such as are seen in states of acute psychotic turmoil.

B. At least five of the following symptoms are required to have appeared as part of the episode for definite and four for probable (for past episodes, because of memory difficulty, one less symptom is required).

(1) Poor appetite or weight loss or increased appetite or weight gain (change of 1 lb. a week over several weeks or ten lbs. a year when not dieting).

(2) Sleep difficulty or sleeping too much.

(3) Loss of energy, fatigability, or tiredness.

(4) Psychomotor agitation or retardation (but not mere subjective feeling of restlessness or being slowed down).

(5) Loss of interest or pleasure in usual activities, including social contact or sex (do not include if limited to a period when delusional or hallucinating). (This loss may or may not be pervasive.)

(6) Feelings of self-reproach or excessive or inappropriate guilt (either may be delusional).

(7) Complaints or evidence of diminished ability to think or concentrate, such as slowed thinking, or indecisiveness (do not include if associated with marked formal thought disorder).

(8) Recurrent thought of death or suicide, or any suicidal behavior.

C. Duration of dysphoric features of at least one week beginning with the first noticeable change in the subject's usual condition (definite if lasted more than two weeks, probable if one to two weeks).

D. Sought or was referred for help from someone during the dysphoric period, took medication, or had impairment in functioning with family, at home, at school, at work, or socially.

E. None of the following which suggest Schizophrenia is present:

(1) Delusions of being controlled (or influenced), or of thought broadcasting, insertion, or withdrawal.

(2) Non-affective hallucinations of any type throughout the day for several days or intermittently throughout a one week period.

(3) Auditory hallucinations in which either a voice keeps up a running commentary on the subject's behaviors or thoughts as they occur, or two or more voices converse with each other.

(4) At some time during the period of illness had more than one month when he exhibited no prominent depressive symptoms but had delusions or hallucinations (although typical depressive delusions such as delusions of guilt, sin, poverty, nihilism, or self-deprecation, or hallucinations with similar content are not included).

(5) Preoccupation with a delusion or hallucination to the relative exclusion of other symptoms or concerns (other than typical depressive delusions of guilt, sin, poverty, nihilism, self-deprecation or hallucinations with similar content).

(6) Definite instances of marked formal thought disorder (as defined in this manual (Spitzer *et al.*, 1978*b*), accompanied by either blunted or inappropriate affect, delusions or hallucinations of any type, or grossly disorganized behavior.

F. Does not meet the criteria for Schizophrenia, Residual subtype (see Chapter B8.)

Subtypes of major depressive disorder

This section is primarily for studies in which there is interest in one or more subtypes of Major Depressive Disorder. The diagnoses in this section describe different ways of categorizing such subjects who meet the criteria for Probable or Definite Major Depressive Disorder, and therefore many subjects will meet the criteria for several categories. *Probable* in this section refers to the subtype, not the certainty that the condition meets the criteria for Major Depressive Disorder.

a. Primary major depressive disorder

The first appearance of probable or definite Major Depressive Disorder was not preceded by any of the following (either probable or definite) although these conditions may have occurred afterwards: Schizophrenia, Schizo-affective Disorder, Panic Disorder, Phobic Disorder, Obsessive Compulsive Disorder, Briquet's Disorder (Somatization Disorder), Anti-social Personality, Alcoholism, Drug Use Disorder, or Preferential Homosexuality. Episodes of Manic Disorder or Hypomanic Disorder may or may not have been present.

b. Secondary major depressive disorder

A period of Major Depressive Disorder (either probable or definite) was preceded by any of the conditions listed below (either probable or definite). (Note: It is possible for a subject to have had both Primary and Secondary Major Depressive Disorders, for example, depression at age 20 and 40 and Alcoholism beginning at age 30 and another depressive episode later.) Another category, Depressive Syndrome Superimposed on Residual Schizophrenia, is also a type of Secondary Depression. Check the condition(s) which existed prior to the development of Secondary Major Depressive Disorder.

—Schizophrenia (with full remission)
—Obsessive Compulsive Disorder
—Phobic disorder
—Antisocial Personality
—Drug Use Disorder
—Schizo-affective Disorder
—Panic Disorder

—Briquet's Disorder (Somatization Disorder)
—Alcoholism
—Preferential Homosexuality (not limited to discrete periods of life)
—Anorexia
—Transsexualism
—Organic Brain Syndrome

The St. Louis group no longer makes a diagnosis of Secondary Depression because of a pre-existing life-threatening condition.

c. Recurrent unipolar major depressive disorder

This is for individuals who have *never* met the criteria for Manic Disorder, Hypomanic Disorder, or Schizo-affective Disorder, Manic Type but who have had two or more episodes that met the criteria for probable or definite Major Depressive Disorder each separated by at least two months of return to more or less usual functioning.

d. Psychotic major depressive disorder

This category is considered for all subjects who have had a Major Depressive Disorder (either probable or definite).

Note: The term Psychotic Depressive Reaction in the standard nomenclature often involves the additional concepts of severity of functional impairment and endogenous phenomena which are not included in this category and are covered separately in other subtypes. This category here is not used in the sense of a psychotic–neurotic dichotomy and thus there is no implication that subjects not so classified thereby have a neurotic depression. (Note: The only delusional or hallucinating subjects who would be considered here are those who do not meet the criteria for Schizo-affective Disorder.)

Either A or B is required.

A. Delusions
B. Hallucinations

e. Incapacitating major depressive disorder

This category is considered for all subjects who have had a probable or definite Major Depressive Disorder. It is applied to subjects who might be classified as Psychotic Depressive Reaction in the standard nomenclature on the basis of extreme severity of functional impairment.

Because of severity of depressive symptoms, the subject is unable to carry out *any* relatively complex goal directed activity such as work, taking care of the house, or sustaining attention and participation in social or recreational activities, i.e., hobbies, reading, going to the movies. Do not count if due to refusal or lack of motivation to do the tasks. (If hospitalized, the impairment in functioning should such be   such that the patient obviously could not carry out the activities if given a chance to do so.)

f. Endogenous major depressive disorder

This category is considered for all subjects with a current episode that meets the criteria for probable or definite Major Depressive Disorder. It is applied to those subjects who show a particular symptom picture that many research studies indicate is associated with good response to somatic therapy. Ignore the presence or absence of precipitating events even though this feature is often associated with the term 'endogenous.'

From groups A and B a total of at least four symptoms for probable, six for definite, including at least one symptom from group A.

A. (1) Distinct quality of depressed mood, i.e., depressed mood is perceived as distinctly different from the kind of feeling he would have or has had following the death of a loved one.
   (2) Lack of reactivity to environmental changes (once depressed doesn't feel better, even temporarily, when something good happens).
   (3) Mood is regularly worse in the morning.
   (4) Pervasive loss of interest or pleasure.

B. (1) Feelings of self-reproach or excessive or inappropriate guilt.
   (2) Early morning awakening or middle insomnia.
   (3) Psychomotor retardation or agitation (more than mere subjective feeling of being slowed down or restless).
   (4) Poor appetite.
   (5) Weight loss (two lbs. a week over several weeks or 20 lbs. in a year when not dieting).
   (6) Loss of interest or pleasure (may or may not be pervasive) in usual activities or decreased sexual drive.

g. Agitated major depressive disorder

This category is considered for all subjects with a current episode that meets the criteria for probable or definite Major Depressive Disorder. At least two of the following manifestations of psychomotor agitation (not merely subjective anxiety) are required for *several* days during the current episode:

(1) Pacing.
(2) Handwringing.
(3) Unable to sit still.
(4) Pulling or rubbing on hair, skin, clothing, or other objects.
(5) Outbursts of complaining or shouting.
(6) Talks on and on or can't seem to stop talking.

h. Retarded major depressive disorder

This category is considered for all subjects with a current episode that meets the criteria for probable or definite Major Depressive Disorder. At least two of the following manifestations of psychomotor retardation are required *for at least one week* during the current episode:

(1) Slowed speech.
(2) Increased pauses before answering.
(3) Low or monotonous speech.
(4) Mute or markedly decreased amount of speech.
(5) Slowed body movements.

i. Situational major depressive disorder

This category is considered for all subjects with a current episode that meets the criteria for a probable or definite Major Depressive Disorder. It is applied to those subjects in whom the depressive illness has developed after an event or in a situation that seems likely to have contributed to the appearance of the episode at that time. In making this judgment consider the amount of stress inherent in the event or situation, the cumulative effect of such stresses, and the closeness of the events to the onset or exacerbation of the depressive episode.

Definite is for situations in which the episode almost certainly would not have developed at that time, in the absence of the external events.

Example: Depressive episode immediately following the sudden death of a loved one. Probable is for situations in which the episode probably would not have developed at that time, in the absence of the external events.

Example: Depressive episode several months after increasing business difficulties.

j. Simple major depressive disorder

This category is considered for all subjects with a current episode that meets the criteria for probable or definite Major Depressive Disorder. It is applied to depressive episodes that develop in a person who has shown no significant signs of psychiatric disturbance in the year prior to the development of the current episode, with the exception of symptomatology associated with either Major or Minor Depressive Disorder, Manic or Hypomanic Disorder.

Often depressive episodes begin with symptoms other than those in the classic depressive syndrome, such as phobias, panic attacks, or excessive somatic concerns. In such instances, these symptoms should be regarded as part of the depressive episode unless the duration of the other symptoms is sufficient to warrant a separate diagnosis.

Note: The concept of Simple Major Depressive Disorder is not identical with the concept of Primary Major Depressive Disorder. An individual who had Alcoholism followed by more than one year of abstinence who then developed a depression would be categorized as having both a Simple and a Secondary Major Depressive Disorder.

COMMENTARY

The research diagnostic criteria (RDC) were developed as part of a collaborative project on the psychobiology of depressive disorders sponsored by the Clinical Research Branch of the National Institute of Mental Health, USA (Maas *et al.*, 1980). They are described as an elaboration and modification of the Feighner criteria (Feighner *et al.*, 1972).

By introducing exclusion criteria and creating new categories such as schizoaffective, the RDC is able to maintain a narrow definition of depression and mania and still classify most patients. Major affective disorders are further subdivided into non-mutually exclusive subtypes to permit testing of many hypotheses relevant to affective illness. The RDC can be used with direct examination or with detailed case records. For further increase of reliability, a structured interview, the Schedule for Affective Disorders and Schizophrenia (SADS) has been developed (Endicott and Spitzer, 1978).

Manic disorders

The diagnostic criteria for mania contain:

(1) Symptomatological criteria (reported symptoms are rated as inclusion criteria **B1**, **B2**, **B5**, and **B7**, and as exclusion criteria **E1–E5**, observed symptoms as inclusion criteria **B6** and **C1**. **A**, **B2**, and **B3** may be reported and/or observed)
(2) Non-symptomatological criteria
    Social functioning (**C2**)
    Hospitalization (**C3**)
    Duration of illness (**D**)

For a diagnosis of manic disorder the following is required: elevated or expansive mood (or irritable mood), at least three (four) of seven symptoms of **B**, signs of a severe overall disturbance (one of **C**), an illness duration of at least one week, and exclusion of criteria which suggest schizophrenia (**E**).

To summarize, the inclusion criteria for this category are almost identical with the Feighner criteria, but the exclusion criteria have been specified in greater detail to differentiate mania from schizoaffective disorder, manic type. Of further importance is the differential diagnosis for hypomanic disorder.

Hypomanic disorder

For a diagnosis of hypomanic disorder, the following is required: elevated, expansive, or irritable mood, at least two of the symptoms noted in manic disorder **B** (three symptoms if mood is only irritable), duration of mood disturbance at least one week for definite diagnosis (probable if two to six days), exclusion of criteria for schizophrenia, schizoaffective disorder, or manic disorder.

This category has been included to facilitate the identification of patients who may have an underlying bipolar affective disorder and may therefore respond differentially to somatic therapy as compared to patients who have had only depressive episodes.

Bipolar depression with mania (bipolar 1)
Bipolar depression with hypomania (bipolar 2)

These criteria include the course of disease in the diagnosis. So, the RDC criteria allow for simultaneous assignment of subjects on the basis of episode diagnosis as well as longitudinal diagnosis. The use of both episode and lifetime diagnoses makes it possible to utilize combinations of information gathered from symptomatology and clinical course.

Major depressive disorder

The diagnostic criteria for major depressive disorder contain the following:

(1) Symptomatological criteria

   (a) Inclusion criteria (**B1**, **B2**, **B3**, **B5**, **B6**, **B7**, and **B8** are reported criteria; **A** and **B4** are observed and/or reported)
   (b) Exclusion criteria (only reported criteria: E1–E6)

(2) Non-symptomatological criteria

   Duration of illness (**C**) and treatment or impairment in functioning (**D**)

For a diagnosis of major depressive disorder the following is required: dysphoric mood or pervasive loss of interest or pleasure; at least five of eight symptoms of **B**; duration of illness of at least two weeks (one week for probable diagnosis); a certain amount of impairment; the exclusion of symptoms which suggest schizophrenia; and the exclusion of criteria for schizophrenia, residual subtype (see Chapter B8).

Jaspers' (1963) hierarchical principle cannot be applied, for if there are symptoms of schizophrenic as well as affective disorders, the criteria for schizoaffective disorder will be fulfilled in most cases.

All the conditions in the RDC (with the exception of alcoholism, drug use disorder, and other psychiatric disorder) are to be diagnosed only when there is no known organic etiology for the symptoms.

To summarize, the category of major depressive disorder includes some cases which would be categorized as neurotic depression and virtually all which would be classified as psychotic depression and manic depressive illness, depressed type.

The Feighner criteria and RDC are quite similar, although several important differences exist: whereas the Feighner criteria require dysphoric mood, the RDC recognize either dysphoric mood or a pervasive loss of interest in pleasure. The RDC drop 'fearful' and 'worried' as acceptable dysphoric moods and accept weight gain as well as weight loss as a depressive symptom. The exclusion criteria are specified in much greater detail in the RDC than in the Feighner criteria to facilitate the differential diagnosis with schizoaffective disorder. Other differential diagnoses to be considered are minor depressive disorder, intermittent depressive disorder, cyclothymic personality, and labile personality. Patients who meet the criteria for probable or definite major depressive disorder are further subdivided into a number of non-mutually exclusive categories:

Primary/secondary major depressive disorder

The definition of primary major depressive disorder is the same as that of the Feighner criteria, i.e., a period of major depressive disorder that had not been preceded by any one in the specific list of non-affective disorders. In contrast, secondary major depressive disorder is defined as a period of major depressive disorder that was preceded by one of the specified disorders.

The problems of this dichotomy are discussed by van Praag (1982).

Simple major depressive disorder

Similar to primary major depressive disorder, only the absence of non-affective disorder is limited to the year prior to the development of the current episode.

Recurrent unipolar depressive disorder

In the RDC, defined as two or more episodes of major depressive disorder, without an episode of manic disorder, hypomanic disorder, or schizoaffective disorder, manic type.

Psychotic major depressive disorder

This term includes all patients with a major depressive disorder and evidence of delusions or hallucinations.

Endogenous major depressive disorder

The term 'endogenous' is reserved for a separate class of patients who manifest the constellation of vegetative symptoms and biorhythmical changes regardless of the presence or absence of precipitating events.

Problems of the taxonomy of this definition are discussed by Williams and Spitzer (1982).

Incapacitating major depressive disorder

Defined by the judgment of severe impairment in functioning.

Situational major depressive disorder

This class is for patients who develop a major depressive disorder after an event or in a situation that seems likely to have contributed to the appearance of the episode at the time.

DSM-III does not use this concept as a basis for subdividing major depressive disorder because of the lack of evidence that major depressive disorders which have been precipitated by stress differ from those which were not in terms of premorbid personality, response to somatic treatment, long-term outcome, and family history (Williams and Spitzer 1982). On the other hand, there is some evidence that this distinction has some predictive value for psychotherapy (Prusoff *et al.*, 1980).

Agitated and retarded major depressive disorder

These terms are used to classify patients with major depressive disorder who show a disturbance in psychomotor functioning for several days during an episode of illness.

C7

Diagnostic and statistical manual of mental disorders, third edition (DSM–III)

Major affective disorders

I. Diagnosis of episode

Manic episode

Diagnostic criteria.

A. One or more distinct periods with a predominantly elevated, expansive, or irritable mood. The elevated or irritable mood must be a prominent part of the illness and relatively persistent, although it may alternate or intermingle with depressive mood.

B. Duration of at least one week (or any duration if hospitalization is necessary), during which, for most of the time, at least three of the following symptoms have persisted (four if the mood is only irritable) and have been present to a significant degree:

   (1) increase in activity (either socially, at work, or sexually) or physical restlessness

   (2) more talkative than usual or pressure to keep talking

   (3) flight of ideas or subjective experience that thoughts are racing

   (4) inflated self-esteem (grandiosity, which may be delusional)

   (5) decreased need for sleep

   (6) distractibility, i.e., attention too easily drawn to unimportant or irrelevant external stimuli

   (7) excessive involvement in activities that have a high potential for painful consequences which is not recognized, e.g., buying sprees, sexual indiscretions, foolish business investments, reckless driving

Source of criteria: Diagnostic and statistical manual of mental disorders, third edition (DSM–III) (1980). Washington, DC: American Psychiatric Association.

C. Neither of the following dominate the clinical picture when an affective syndrome (i.e., criteria A and B above) is not present, that is, before it developed or after it has remitted:

 (1) preoccupation with a mood-incongruent delusion or hallucination (see definition below)
 (2) bizarre behavior

D. Not superimposed on either Schizophrenia, Schizophreniform Disorder, or a Paranoid Disorder.
E. Not due to any Organic Mental Disorder, such as Substance Intoxication.

(*Note:* A hypomanic episode is a pathological disturbance similar to, but not as severe as, a manic episode.)

Fifth-digit code numbers and criteria for subclassification of manic episode:

6 – In Remission. This fifth-digit category should be used when in the past the individual met the full criteria for a manic episode but now is essentially free of manic symptoms or has some signs of the disorder but does not meet the full criteria. The differentiation of this diagnosis from no mental disorder requires consideration of the period of time since the last episode, the number of previous episodes, and the need for continued evaluation or prophylactic treatment.

4 – With Psychotic Features. This fifth-digit category should be used when there apparently is gross impairment in reality testing, as when there are delusions or hallucinations or grossly bizarre behavior. When possible specify whether the psychotic features are mood-congruent or mood-incongruent. (The non-ICD-9-CM fifth-digit 7 may be used instead to indicate that the psychotic features are mood-incongruent; otherwise, mood-congruence may be assumed.) Mood-congruent Psychotic Features: Delusions or hallucinations whose content is entirely consistent with the themes of inflated worth, power, knowledge, identity, or special relationship to a deity or famous person; flight of ideas without apparent awareness by the individual that the speech is not understandable.
Mood-incongruent Psychotic Features: Either (*a*) or (*b*):

 (*a*) Delusions or hallucinations whose content does not involve themes of either inflated worth, power, knowledge, identity, or special relationship to a deity or famous person. Included are such symptoms as persecutory delusions, thought insertion, and delusions of being controlled, whose content has no apparent relationship to any of the themes noted above.
 (*b*) Any of the following catatonic symptoms: stupor, mutism, negativism, posturing.

2 – Without Psychotic Features. Meets the criteria for manic episode, but no psychotic features are present.
0 – Unspecified.

Major depressive episode

Diagnostic criteria

A. Dysphoric mood or loss of interest or pleasure in all or almost all usual activities and pastimes. The dysphoric mood is characterized by symptoms such as the following: depressed, sad, blue, hopeless, low, down in the dumps, irritable. The mood disturbance must be prominent and relatively persistent, but not necessarily the most dominant symptom, and does not include momentary shifts from one dysphoric mood to another dysphoric mood, e.g., anxiety to depression to anger, such as are seen in states of acute psychotic turmoil. (For children under six, dysphoric mood may have to be inferred from a persistently sad facial expression.)

B. At least four of the following symptoms have each been present nearly every day for a period of at least two weeks (in children under six, at least three of the first four):

(1) poor appetite or significant weight loss (when not dieting) or increased appetite or significant weight gain (in children under six consider failure to make expected weight gains)
(2) insomnia or hypersomnia
(3) psychomotor agitation or retardation (but not merely subjective feelings of restlessness or being slowed down) (in children under six, hypoactivity)
(3) loss of interest or pleasure in usual activities, or decrease in sexual drive not limited to a period when delusional or hallucinating (in children under six, signs of apathy)
(5) loss of energy: fatigue
(6) feelings of worthlessness, self-reproach, or excessive or inappropriate guilt (either may be delusional)
(7) complaints or evidence of diminished ability to think or concentrate, such as slowed thinking, or indecisiveness not associated with marked loosening of associations or incoherence
(8) recurrent thoughts of death, suicidal ideation, wishes to be dead, or suicide attempt

C. Neither of the following dominate the clinical picture when an affective syndrome (i.e., criteria A and B above) is not present, that is, before it developed or after it has remitted:

(1) preoccupation with a mood-incongruent delusion or hallucination (see definition below)

(2) bizarre behavior

D. Not superimposed on either Schizophrenia, Schizophreniform Disorder, or a Paranoid Disorder.

E. Not due to any Organic Mental Disorder or Uncomplicated Bereavement.

Fifth-digit code numbers and criteria for subclassification of major depressive episode:

(When psychotic features and melancholia are present the coding system requires that the clinician record the single most clinically significant characteristic.)

6 – In Remission. This fifth-digit category should be used when in the past the individual met the full criteria for a major depressive episode but now is essentially free of depressive symptoms or has some signs of the disorder but does not meet the full criteria.

4 – With Psychotic Features. This fifth-digit category should be used when there apparently is gross impairment in reality testing, as when there are delusions or hallucinations, or depressive stupor (the individual is mute and unresponsive). When possible specify whether the psychotic features are mood-congruent or mood-incongruent. (The non-ICD-9-CM fifth-digit 7 may be used instead to indicate that the psychotic features are mood-incongruent; otherwise, mood-congruence may be assumed.)

Mood-congruent Psychotic Features. Delusions or hallucinations whose content is entirely consistent with the themes of either personal inadequacy, guilt, disease, death, nihilism, or deserved punishment; depressive stupor (the individual is mute and unresponsive).

Mood-incongruent Psychotic Features. Delusions or hallucinations whose content does not involve themes of either personal inadequacy, guilt, disease, death, nihilism, or deserved punishment. Included here are such symptoms as persecutory delusions, thought insertion, thought broadcasting, and delusions of control, whose content has no apparent relationship to any of the themes noted above.

3 – With Melancholia. Loss of pleasure in all or almost all activities, lack of reactivity to usually pleasurable stimuli (doesn't feel much better, even temporarily, when something good happens), and at least three of the following:

(a) distinct quality of depressed mood, i.e., the depressed mood is perceived as distinctly different from the kind of feeling experi-

enced following the death of a loved one
  (b) the depression is regularly worse in the morning
  (c) early morning awakening (at least two hours before usual time of awakening)
  (d) marked psychomotor retardation or agitation
  (e) significant anorexia or weight loss
  (f) excessive or inappropriate guilt

2 – Without Melancholia
0 – Unspecified

II. Diagnosis of illness

Bipolar disorder

296.6x Bipolar disorder, mixed

Diagnostic criteria

Use fifth-digit coding for manic episode.

A. Current (or most recent) episode involves the full symptomatic picture of both manic and major depressive episodes, intermixed or rapidly alternating every few days.
B. Depressive symptoms are prominent and last at least a full day.

296.4x Bipolar disorder, manic

Diagnostic criterion

Currently (or most recently) in a manic episode. (If there has been a previous manic episode, the current episode need not meet the full criteria for a manic episode.)

296.5x Bipolar disorder, depressed

Diagnostic criteria

A. Has had one or more manic episodes.
B. Currently (or most recently) in a major depressive episode. (If there has been a previous major depressive episode, the current episode of depression need not meet the full criteria for a major depressive episode.)

Major depression

296.2x Major depression, single episode

296.3x Major depression, recurrent

Diagnostic criteria

A. One or more major depressive episodes.
B. Has never had a manic episode.

COMMENTARY

The most important issues with respect to the clinical logic behind DSM–III's approach – using inclusion and exclusion criteria – for defining and diagnosing different forms of so-called endogenous psychotic illness were exemplified on the basis of the discussions of DSM–III schizophrenic, schizophreniform and brief reactive psychotic disorders in Chapter B9 and will not be repeated here. In particular, the central role of 'full' affective syndromes as an exclusion criterion in diagnosing these illnesses was fully considered there.

Many similarities exist between the Feighner, RDC and DSM–III concepts of major affective disorder (see Chapters C5, C6 and C7) because the so-called 'affective' inclusion items found in criteria A and B in all three diagnostic systems are practically identical. Moreover, the same is true for their chronological inclusion criteria; these require about one to two weeks for a manic episode (criterion C in the Feighner and D in the RDC systems, and part of criterion B in DSM–III) and one to four weeks for a major depressive episode (criterion C in the Feighner and RDC systems, and part of criterion B in DSM–III).

There are, however, some important differences between the Feighner, RDC and DSM–III definitions of major affective disorder. For example, the exclusion symptom criteria of the RDC preclude a diagnosis of affective disorder when 'contamination' with so-called 'schizophrenic' or mood-incongruent symptoms has occurred, whereas the Feighner definition in this regard sets no such limits. In contrast, however, DSM–III places only minimal limitations on the allowable presence of these 'schizophrenic' or mood-incongruent features when they manifest themselves as part of a 'full' affective syndrome; indeed, DSM–III states clearly that the diagnosis of a major affective episode can still be made in the presence of 'schizophrenic' or mood-incongruent elements provided they do not appear prior to the development of, or after the passing of, a 'full' affective syndrome and provided that, in such instances, they do not dominate the clinical picture. Obviously, DSM–III's rules of application in this area are more or less the reverse of its rule governing the relationships between 'schizophrenic' symptoms and 'full' affective syndromes in its definitions of schizophrenic, schizophreniform and brief reactive psychotic disorders.

A few other diagnostic innovations in DSM–III's concept of major affective disorder also deserve mention. Although explicit criteria for a manic episode are given in DSM–III, there is no category of mania as such. In other words, the first time a DSM–III manic episode is diagnosed, the illness is called bipolar disorder from that point on, irrespective of whether the patient ever had a DSM–III major depressive episode in the past or ever will have one in the future. A DSM–III major affective disorder can be diagnosed only providing that a DSM–III schizophrenic disorder has never occurred in the past; should the criteria for a 'full' affective syndrome occur in such a situation – e.g., a superimposed 'full' affective syndrome on DSM–III schizophrenic disorder during a non-'psychotic' segment of illness – it is classified as atypical affective disorder.

The last paragraph of the commentary on DSM–III schizophrenic, schizophreniform, and brief reactive psychotic disorders in Chapter B9 focused specifically on the clinical rationale involved in comparisons with other diagnostic systems such as the Feighner and RDC. On the basis of these conclusions one can argue perhaps that DSM–III major affective disorder might be viewed as being much wider than the corresponding definition of this disorder in the RDC, on the one hand, yet somewhat narrower than that represented by the Feighner concept, on the other.

C8

Diagnostic and statistical manual of mental disorders, third edition, revised (DSM–III–R)

In this section, criteria are provided for Manic and Major Depressive Episodes. These are followed by criteria for the specific mood disorders.

Manic episode

Note: A 'Manic Syndrome' is defined as including criteria A, B, and C below. A 'Hypomanic Syndrome' is defined as including criteria A and B, but not C, i.e., no marked impairment.

A. A distinct period of abnormally and persistently elevated, expansive, or irritable mood.

B. During the period of mood disturbance, at lease three of the following symptoms have persisted (four if the mood is only irritable) and have been present to a significant degree:

    (1) inflated self-esteem or grandiosity

    (2) decreased need for sleep, e.g., feels rested after only three hours of sleep

    (3) more talkative than usual or pressure to keep talking

    (4) flight of ideas or subjective experience that thoughts are racing

    (5) distractibility, i.e., attention too easily drawn to unimportant or irrelevant external stimuli

    (6) increase in goal-directed activity (either socially, at work or school, or sexually) or psychomotor agitation

    (7) excessive involvement in pleasurable activities which have a high potential for painful consequences, e.g., the person engages in

Source of criteria: Diagnostic and statistical manual of mental disorders, third edition, revised (DSM–III–R) (1987). Washington, DC: American Psychiatric Association.

unrestrained buying sprees, sexual indiscretions, or foolish business investments

C. Mood disturbance sufficiently severe to cause marked impairment in occupational functioning or in usual social activities or relationships with others, or to necessitate hospitalization to prevent harm to self or others.
D. At no time during the disturbance have there been delusions or hallucinations for as long as two weeks in the absence of prominent mood symptoms (i.e., before the mood symptoms developed or after they have remitted).
E. Not superimposed on Schizophrenia, Schizophreniform Disorder, Delusional Disorder, or Psychotic Disorder NOS.
F. It cannot be established that an organic factor initiated and maintained the disturbance. **Note:** Somatic antidepressant treatment (e.g., drugs, ECT) that apparently precipitates a mood disturbance should not be considered an etiologic organic factor.

Manic episode codes: fifth-digit code numbers and criteria for severity of current state of bipolar disorder, manic or mixed:

1 – Mild: Meets minimum symptom criteria for a Manic Episode (or almost meets symptom criteria if there has been a previous Manic Episode).
2 – Moderate: Extreme increase in activity or impairment in judgment.
3 – Severe, without Psychotic Features: Almost continual supervision required in order to prevent physical harm to self or others.
4 – With Psychotic Features: Delusions, hallucinations, or catatonic symptoms. If possible, *specify* whether the psychotic features are **mood-congruent** or **mood-incongruent**.

Mood-congruent psychotic features: Delusions or hallucinations whose content is entirely consistent with the typical manic themes of inflated worth, power, knowledge, identity, or special relationship to a deity or famous person.

Mood-incongruent psychotic features: Either (*a*) or (*b*):

(*a*) Delusions or hallucinations whose content does *not* involve the typical manic themes of inflated worth, power, knowledge, identity, or special relationship to a deity or famous person. Included are such symptoms as persecutory delusions (not directly related to grandiose ideas or themes), thought insertion, and delusions of being controlled.
(*b*) Catatonic symptoms, e.g., stupor, mutism, negativism, posturing.

5 – In Partial Remission: Full criteria were previously, but are not currently, met; some signs or symptoms of the disturbance have persisted.

6 – In Full Remission: Full criteria were previously met, but there have been no significant signs or symptoms of the disturbance for at least six months.

0 – Unspecified.

Major depressive episode

Note: A 'Major Depressive Syndrome' is defined as criterion A below.

A. At least five of the following symptoms have been present during the same two-week period and represent a change from previous functioning; at least one of the symptoms is either (1) depressed mood, or (2) loss of interest or pleasure. (Do not include symptoms that are clearly due to a physical condition, mood-incongruent delusions or hallucinations, incoherence, or marked loosening of associations.)

(1) depressed mood (or can be irritable mood in children and adolescents) most of the day, nearly every day, as indicated either by subjective account or observation by others

(2) markedly diminished interest or pleasure in all, or almost all, activities most of the day, nearly every day (as indicated either by subjective account or observation by others of apathy most of the time)

(3) significant weight loss or weight gain when not dieting (e.g., more than 5% of body weight in a month), or decrease or increase in appetite nearly every day (in children, consider failure to make expected weight gains)

(4) insomnia or hypersomnia nearly every day

(5) psychomotor agitation or retardation nearly every day (observable by others, not merely subjective feelings of restlessness or being slowed down)

(6) fatigue or loss of energy nearly every day

(7) feelings of worthlessness or excessive or inappropriate guilt (which may be delusional) nearly every day (not merely self-reproach or guilt about being sick)

(8) diminished ability to think or concentrate, or indecisiveness, nearly every day (either by subjective account or as observed by others)

(9) recurrent thoughts of death (not just fear of dying), recurrent suicidal ideation without a specific plan, or a suicide attempt or a specific plan for committing suicide

B. (1) It cannot be established that an organic factor initiated and maintained the disturbance

    (2) The disturbance is not a normal reaction to the death of a loved one (Uncomplicated Bereavement)

    Note: Morbid preoccupation with worthlessness, suicidal ideation, marked functional impairment or psychomotor retardation, or prolonged duration suggest bereavement complicated by Major Depression.

C. At no time during the disturbance have there been delusions or hallucinations for as long as two weeks in the absence of prominent mood symptoms (i.e., before the mood symptoms developed or after they have remitted).

D. Not superimposed on Schizophrenia, Schizophreniform Disorder, Delusional Disorder, or Psychotic Disorder NOS.

Major depressive episode codes: fifth-digit code numbers and criteria for severity of current state of bipolar disorder, depressed, or major depression:

    1 – **Mild:** Few, if any, symptoms in excess of those required to make the diagnosis, *and* symptoms result in only minor impairment in occupational functioning or in usual social activities or relationships with others.

    2 – **Moderate:** Symptoms or functional impairment between 'mild' and 'severe.'

    3 – **Severe, without Psychotic Features:** Several symptoms in excess of those required to make the diagnosis, *and* symptoms markedly interfere with occupational functioning or with usual social activities or relationships with others.

    4 – **With Psychotic Features:** Delusions or hallucinations. If possible, *specify* whether the psychotic features are **mood-congruent** or **mood-incongruent**.

    Mood-congruent psychotic features: Delusions or hallucinations whose content is entirely consistent with the typical depressive themes of personal inadequacy, guilt, disease, death, nihilism, or deserved punishment.

    Mood-incongruent psychotic features: Delusions or hallucinations whose content does *not* involve typical depressive themes of personal inadequacy, guilt, disease, death, nihilism, or deserved punishment. Included here are such symptoms as persecutory delusions (not directly related to depressive themes), thought insertion, thought broadcasting, and delusions of control.

    5 – **In Partial Remission:** Intermediate between 'In Full Remission' and 'Mild,' *and* no previous Dysthymia. (If Major Depressive Episode

was superimposed on Dysthymia, the diagnosis of Dysthymia alone is given once the full criteria for a Major Depressive Episode are no longer met.)

6 – **In Full Remission:** During the past six months no significant signs or symptoms of the disturbance.

0 – **Unspecified.**

Specify chronic if current episode has lasted two consecutive years without a period of two month or longer during which there were no significant depressive symptoms.

Specify if current episode is **Melancholic Type.**

Diagnostic criteria for melancholic type

The presence of at least five of the following:

(1) loss of interest or pleasure in all, or almost all, activities
(2) lack of reactivity to usually pleasurable stimuli (does not feel much better, even temporarily, when something good happens)
(3) depression regularly worse in the morning
(4) early morning awakening (at least two hours before usual time of awakening)
(5) psychomotor retardation or agitation (not merely subjective complaints)
(6) significant anorexia or weight loss (e.g., more than 5% of body weight in a month)
(7) no significant personality disturbance before first major depressive episode
(8) one or more previous major depressive episodes followed by complete, or nearly complete, recovery
(9) previous good response to specific and adequate somatic antidepressant therapy, e.g., tricyclics, ECT, MAOI, lithium

Diagnostic criteria for seasonal pattern

A. There has been a regular temporal relationship between the onset of an episode of Bipolar Disorder (including Bipolar Disorder NOS) or Recurrent Major Depression (including Depressive Disorder NOS) and a particular 60-day period of the year (e.g., regular appearance of depression between the beginning of October and the end of November).
Note: Do not include cases in which there is an obvious effect of seasonally related psychosocial stressors, e.g., regularly being unemployed every winter.
B. Full remissions (or a change from depression to mania or hypomania)

also occurred within a particular 60-day period of the year (e.g., depression disappears from mid-February to mid-April).
C. There have been at least three episodes of mood disturbance in three separate years that demonstrated the temporal seasonal relationship defined in A and B; at least two of the years were consecutive.
D. Seasonal episodes of mood disturbance, as described above, outnumbered any nonseasonal episodes of such disturbance that may have occurred by more than three to one.

Bipolar disorders

296.6x Bipolar disorder, mixed

For fifth digit, use the Manic Episode codes [DSM–III–R, p. 126] to describe current state.

A. Current (or most recent) episode involves the full symptomatic picture of both Manic and Major Depressive Episodes (except for the duration requirement of two weeks for depressive symptoms) ([ibid.] p. 125 and p. 128), intermixed or rapidly alternating every few days.
B. Prominent depressive symptoms lasting at least a full day.

Specify if **seasonal pattern** (see p. 131 [ibid.]).

296.4x Bipolar disorder, manic

For fifth digit, use the Manic Episode codes ([ibid.] p. 126) to describe current state.

Currently (or most recently) in a Manic Episode ([ibid.] p. 125). (If there has been a previous Manic Episode, the current episode need not meet the full criteria for a manic episode.)

Specify if **seasonal pattern** (see p. 131 [ibid.]).

296.5x Bipolar disorder, depressed

For fifth digit, use the Major Depressive Episode codes ([ibid.] p. 129) to describe current state.

A. Has had one or more Manic Episodes ([ibid.] p. 125).
B. Currently (or more recently) in a Major Depressive Episode ([ibid.] p. 128). (If there has been a previous Major Depressive Episode, the current episode need not meet the full criteria for a Major Depressive Episode.)

Specify if **seasonal pattern** (see p. 131 [ibid.]).

COMMENTARY

Some important changes have been made in the original DSM–III concept of affective disorders discussed in Chapter C7, and these have been incorporated in a new DSM–III–R definition. In general one notes that the more descriptive term 'mood disorders' has now been adopted, and the classification has been reorganized so that the bipolar disorders (including cyclothymia) and the depressive disorders (major depression and dysthymia) are grouped together.

One of the most important specific changes is that the original A (mood) criterion of the major depressive episode has now been split into its two component parts, namely, dysphoric mood and marked loss of interest or pleasure, and these parts then established as the new A1 and A2 items, respectively; moreover, seven of the original B items now become the new items A3 to A9. However, since either A1 or A2 represents a *sine qua non* requirement of the new definition, and since at least four of the remaining seven items of criterion A must be present for a positive rating, the rules of application seem to be more or less the same as in DSM–III.

Another key change with respect to both the manic and major depressive episode involved the original DSM–III C criterion, which dealt with the relationship between the 'full' affective syndrome and the so-called 'schizophrenic' phenomena of the active phase; this relationship is also defined in the new C criterion for major depressive episode and the new D criterion for the manic episode. Whereas in the original C criterion the presence of bizarre behavior or mood-incongruent delusions/ hallucinations before the appearance of, or after the passing of, a 'full' affective syndrome served as exclusion criteria for major affective disorder, in the new exclusion criterion the types of psychotic phenomena allowed clearly range over a much wider spectrum in the sense that not only mood-incongruent but also mood-congruent delusions or hallucinations now seem to be acceptable. Furthermore, whereas in the original C criterion only clinical symptomatological dominance, without any rigid time frame, is required of the active phase 'schizophrenic' phenomena, the new exclusion criteria state that the active phase phenomena must be present at least for two weeks before being able to serve as an exclusion criterion for major affective disorder. These latter changes may mean that the new exclusion criteria are now more rigorously defined in DSM–III–R affective disorder.

Some other important modifications worthy of being particularly noted are:

(1) the introduction of various grades of the degree of severity for the manic and the major depressive episodes;

(2) the criteria for melancholia have been rearranged in the form of an index of items (including some non-symptoms), no one of which is now a *sine qua non* requirement (in particular, the original 'lack of reactivity' criterion of melancholia has now lost its *sine qua non* status);
(3) there is now also a chronic specification, to be used when the syndrome has persisted, either in partial remission or at criterion level, for over two years.

C9

Present state examination (PSE)/CATEGO system

Class M+. Manic and mixed affective psychoses

The chief symptoms are:

(i) subjective euphoria, or elation on examination,
(ii) ideomotor pressure,
(iii) grandiose ideas,
(iv) grandiose delusions,
(v) flight of ideas,
(vi) overactivity.

The first symptom must be present together with at least one other, in the absence of symptoms from class S+ [see Chapter B13]. A hypomanic subclass can be distinguished. Mixed affective conditions are included.

Class D+. Depressive psychoses

The chief symptoms are:

(i) depressed mood,
(ii) depressive delusions or hallucinations.

Both symptoms must be present, in the absence of symptoms of class S+ or M+. The commonest diagnosis given to patients in this class is ICD 296.2.

Source of criteria: Wing, J. K., Cooper, J. E. and Sartorius, N.: (1974) *Measurement and classification of psychiatric symptoms.* Cambridge: Cambridge University Press. This corresponds to the ninth edition of the present state examination. The tenth edition is currently under way. It will be included in SCAN (schedules for clinical assessment in neuropsychiatry). See Wing *et al.* (1990).

Class R+. Retarded depression

The chief symptoms are:

(i)   depressed mood,
(ii)   retardation,
(iii)   guilt, self-depreciation, etc.
(iv)   agitation.

The first of these symptoms must be present, together with one of the others, in the absence of depressive delusions or other psychotic symptoms.

COMMENTARY

CATEGO is a computer program for allocating psychiatric patients with functional disorders to one of several 'clinical classes' which are intended for use in research and investigations of clinical diagnosis. For a general description and evaluation the reader is referred to Chapter B13 of this volume.

Three of the final nine definite CATEGO classes are relevant for affective psychoses: M (mania and mixed affective psychosis), D (depressive psychoses), and R (retarded depression). Furthermore, a class N (neurotic depression) is defined.

The definition of class M as provided by Wing *et al.* (1974) is complex. Approximately, it requires the presence of elation of mood or subjective euphoria together with at least one other 'manic' symptom – namely, ideomotor pressure, grandiose ideas, grandiose delusions, flight of ideas or overactivity, in the absence of: (1) symptoms of class S+ or S?; (2) a combination of other psychotic symptoms suggesting class P.

The CATEGO system, therefore, follows Karl Jaspers' (1963) hierarchical principle. If the assignment is certain the symbol M+ is used; doubtful combinations are classified as class M?. Since 'mixed affective psychoses' are included in class M of the nine-group classification, obviously a second hierarchical principle has been introduced: mania overrides depression if both are present in the last four weeks before the interview. However, a class for mixed affective psychosis (MAP) is provided in the 50-group classification. Class D is defined by the presence of depressive delusions or hallucinations together with depressed mood. The same two exclusion categories are used as for M and, again, if the assignment is certain the symbol D+ is used and a class D? is provded for doubtful cases.

Class R is referred to as 'retarded depression.' Depressed mood must be present together with retardation, guilt (self-depreciation, etc.), or agitation. No depressive delusions or other psychotic symptoms must be present. In the international pilot study of schizophrenia (IPSS; WHO, 1973) and the US/UK diagnostic project (Cooper *et al.*, 1972), class R+ cases were distributed equally between ICD-8 diagnoses 296.2 (endogenous depression) and 300.4 (depressive neurosis).

Finally, if neither class D+ nor class R+ apply and if a depressed mood is combined with anxiety, the CATEGO program allocates the case to a class N+ ('neurotic depression') or to a class A+ ('anxiety or phobic neurosis') according to the severity and combination of symptoms present.

The distinction between classes D+ and R+, on the one hand, and class N+, on the other, has received some empirical support in life-event and social-network research (Wing and Bebbington, 1982), although contradictory evidence exists (Katschnig, 1984*b*).

C10

Vienna research criteria (endogenomorphic-cyclothymic axial syndrome, Berner)

Endogenomorphic-cyclothymic axial syndrome

A and B obligatory

A. Appearance of marked changes in affectivity, emotional resonance, or drive following a period of habitual functioning.
B. Appearance of biorhythmic disturbances.
     Symptoms 1 and 2 are required:

  1. Diurnal variations of affectivity, emotional resonance, or drive
  2. Sleep disturbances
       (At least one of the following symptoms is required):

    (a) Interrupted sleep   (c) Shortened sleep
    (b) Early awakening   (d) Prolonged sleep

Subtypes

The following 6 subtypes differ only with regard to the specific features of affectivity, emotional resonance and drive listed under A.
   The biorhythmic disturbances as defined under B are the same for all subtypes.
   Consequently the following subtype-criteria refer only to A.

Subtype 1
Endogenomorphic-depressive axial syndrome

A and B obligatory

A. Appearance of marked changes in affectivity, emotional resonance, or drive following a period of habitual functioning.

At least one of the following symptoms is required:

1. Depressive mood (with or without anxiety)
2. Emotional resonance either lacking or limited to depressive responses
3. Reduced drive or agitation

B. Appearance of biorhythmic disturbances as defined in the general endogenomorphic-cyclothymic axial syndrome

Subtype 2
Endogenomorphic-manic axial syndrome

A and B obligatory

A. Appearance of marked changes in affectivity, emotional resonance, or drive following a period of habitual functioning.
   At least one of the following symptoms is required:

1. Euphoric/expansive mood
2. Emotional resonance limited to manic responses
3. Increased drive

B. Appearance of biorhythmic disturbances as defined in the general endogenomorphic-cyclothymic axial syndrome

Subtype 3
Endogenomorphic-dysphoric axial syndrome

A and B obligatory

A. Appearance of marked changes in affectivity, emotional resonance, or drive following a period of habitual functioning.
   At least one of the following symptoms is required:

1. Irritable mood (dysphoria)
2. Emotional resonance limited to hostile responses
3. Increased readines to hostile acting out

B. Appearance of biorhythmic disturbances as defined in the general endogenomorphic-cyclothymic axial syndrome

Subtype 4
Axial syndrome of endogenomorphic anxiety*

A and B obligatory

A. Appearance of marked changes in affectivity and emotional resonance following a period of habitual functioning.
Symptoms 1 and 2 are required:

1. Anxiety states or anxiety attacks
2. Persistent or episodic distractability, startle responses and apprehensiveness

B. Appearance of biorhythmic disturbances as defined in the general endogenomorphic-cyclothymic axial syndrome

Subtype 5
Endogenomorphic axial syndrome of unstable mixed states

A and B obligatory

A. Appearance of rapidly alternating swings in affectivity, emotional resonance, or drive following a period of habitual functioning.
At least one of the following symptoms is required:

1. Rapidly alternating swings between depressive and/or anxious, euphoric/expansive, or hostile mood
2. Rapidly alternating and exaggerated emotional resonance touching various affective states (depressive, anxious, manic, hostile)
3. Rapid change between inhibition, agitation, increased drive, and occasionally aggression.
(The rapid swinging can bring about 'concordant' or 'discordant' changes in affectivity and drive – for example, manic mood combined with decreased drive – because each element may swing in a different rhythm

B. Appearance of biorhythmic disturbances as defined in the general endogenomorphic-cyclothymic axial syndrome

* The formation of the axial syndrome of endogenomorphic anxiety comprises generalized anxiety disorder as well as features that are commonly classified as panic disorder.

Subtype 6
Endogenomorphic axial syndrome of stable mixed states

A and B obligatory

A. Appearance of persisting changes in affectivity, emotional resonance, or drive following a period of habitual functioning.
    Symptoms 1 or 2 (or 1 and 2) and 3 are required:

    1. Depressed, anxious, euphoric/expansive or hostile mood
    2. Emotional resonance either lacking in or limited to depressive, manic, hostile or anxious responses
    3. Persistent presence of a drive state contradictory to the mood state and/or the emotional resonance

B. Appearance of biorhythmic disturbances as defined in the general endogenomorphic-cyclothymic axial syndrome

COMMENTARY

The reasons leading to the formulation of the Vienna research criteria and the history of their development have been dealt with already in the discussion on the endogenomorphic-schizophrenic axial syndrome (see Chapter B14); in this connection, special reference was made also to the concept of basic dynamic constellations (Janzarik 1959) and the research on unstable mixed states (Mentzos, 1967). Consideration of these two concepts, and the opinion (Specht, 1901) that dysphoric states as well as certain anxiety states (Sheehan *et al.*, 1980) could constitute special forms of affective psychosis, led to the formulation of an 'endogenomorphic-cyclothymic' axial syndrome* comprising the essential common features of its six subtypes. This decision was based on the following assumptions:

(1) Endogenous cyclothymia occurs not only in the form of typical depressive or manic phases; it can also take on the form of dysphoria, anxiety states, 'unstable mixed states' (rapidly alternating changes in affectivity, emotional resonance and drive) or stable mixed states.
(2) Dynamic derailments, as formulated by Janzarik (ibid.), underlie all these manifestations of cyclothymia; depression, mania, dysphoria, and stable mixed states are stable derailments; unstable mixed states and anxiety states are labile derailments corresponding to the notion of 'dynamic instability.'

---

* The term 'cyclothymic' is used as a synomym for affective disorders of supposed genetic origin.

(3) Since all dynamic derailments are nosologically non-specific, they can be rated only as expressions of affective psychoses when additional criteria make their presence probable. If one wishes to make a cross-sectional diagnosis and spare oneself reliance on genetic information and response to therapy for validation, one must at present rely on appearance of disturbance in affectivity, emotional resonance, and drive (A) coupled with biorhythmic modifications (B) (following a period of habitual functioning).

All six endogenomorphic-cyclothymic axial syndromes are based exclusively on symtomatological criteria. 'Appearance' does not necessarily imply 'abrupt': the symptoms may also develop slowly and progressively; the sole stipulation is that a clear deviation from the habitual state must occur.

The group A symptoms must be felt by the patient or significant others to represent a pronounced change, which is why the word 'marked' qualifies them. This states at the same time that the changes may also be purely qualitative ones: with this definition, for example, depressive phases will be identified both when they occur in a person who has been subdepressed all his life and when they represent something new for someone previously normal or hypomanic. Experience has shown that modifications in sleep behavior and diurnal variations (B) may sometimes appear discretely; in order to apply, they need only represent a change from the usual state. Disclosure in the subtype A1 (mood) relies upon the patient's portrayal; all other criteria are given positive ratings when they are observed as well as when they are reported.

Of the subtype symptoms in group A, only one is required for diagnosis. Therefore, for the diagnosis of cyclothymia the presence of mood abnormalities is not obligatory. The specific formulation of symptom A2 in each of the axial syndromes comes from the experience that emotional responsiveness in stable dynamic derailments and in anxiety states – as long as they are preserved – corresponds to the tone set by the state of affectivity; in the unstable mixed states, however, it can change quickly and excessively in various directions. The symptoms of group A are specified for each of the particular syndromes. The biorhythmic disturbances listed under B are common to all the six subtypes.

Opinion in the literature concerning the frequency and diagnostic value of diurnal variations is divided (Waldmann, 1972; Stallone *et al.*, 1973; Papousek, 1975); nevertheless, they were included in the group B symptoms. The reason for this is founded on the theoretical assumption that the required biorhythmic variations are 'fundamental' disturbances of the endogenous cyclothymias. They may also occur in impairment of brain function of organic or toxic origin but not in disorders of purely psychogenic origin. Experience has shown that diurnal variations, noticed in earlier stages, are often not lived or observed at the acme of the phase. In such cases they are rated as present when either the patient or significant others report them as having lasted in the same form for at least five days within the last four weeks required by present state examination (PSE) (see Chapter C9). Restricting the meaning of diurnal variations to matinal aggravation was waived because other patterns also have often been observed in cyclothymic disorders (such as evening, or morning and evening aggravation of symptoms). Diurnal variations often manifest themselves either in generalized anxiety states, through an aggravation of startle response and vegetative lability during certain times of the day, or, in the case of anxiety attacks, through an increased attack frequency (e.g., 'nocturnal panic attacks'). Only a few comments concerning the bio-rhythmic variations are necessary in this respect: diurnal variations are required for all subtypes. This contrasts with the opinion of many authors who assert that diurnal variations do not manifest themselves in derailments other than depression.

The endogenomorphic-cyclothymic axial syndromes contain no excluding criteria. The gathering of data is accomplished by means of a broadened version of the PSE.

The Vienna criteria for the diagnosis of cyclothymia are theoretical in that they are oriented to the concept of basic dynamic constellations and take biorhythmic variations to the 'fundamental disturbances.' The former is split up into six axial syndromes, which takes into account the hypothesis of the various types of dynamic derailment (Janzarik, 1959; Berner, 1969). The hypothesis of endogeny is reflected in the choice and combination of criteria used in the formulation of the particular axial syndromes: these are made up of symptoms which are deemed to be characteristic for endogenous affective psychoses. This qualification, aside from the theoretically justified application of biorhythmic disturbances, is founded on the experience that the symptoms in question are valid as criteria for attribution to endogenous disorders (Baillarger, 1854; Kraepelin, 1913; Sandifer *et al.*, 1966; Mentzos, 1967; Klerman, 1972; Nutzinger, 1991). Consequently, the particular symptoms constituting the various cyclothymic axial syndromes represent empirical elements.

Non-symptomatological prognosis indicators were not considered, above all because one of the purposes in applying the Vienna research criteria is to find out whether the various constituting symptoms really enable the prediction of an intermittent course. Genetic information was not included in the instrument because it serves also the purpose of validation. The numerous declarations found in the literature that endogenic-cyclothymic phases often can be triggered by life events (Tölle, 1980) underlie the decision not to include the presence or absence of life events in the Vienna cyclothymia criteria. The presence of the group B biorhythmic disturbances is considered to exclude purely psychogenic disturbances. Demarcation to schizophrenia as in the hierarchical principle (Jaspers, 1963) is not undertaken: in the presence of both the endogenomorphic-cyclothymic axial syndrome and the schizophrenic axial syndrome (see Chapter B14) a 'schizoaffective syndrome' is diagnosed. Organically or toxically caused symptoms exclude attribution to one of the endogenomorphic-cyclothymic axial syndromes from the very start.

Individually considered, the endogenomorphic-depressive and endogenomorphic-manic axial syndromes are conceived more narrowly than the criteria for depression and mania of other authors because they require the presence of biorhythmic changes B1 and B2. The group of cyclothymias taken as a whole is broadened considerably, on the one hand, by the concept of endogenous anxiety, and, on the other hand, at the expense of attribution to schizophrenia through the inclusion of dysphoric derailments and unstable and stable mixed states. The Vienna criteria do not contain the assumption that cyclothymia is necessarily an illness entity; they leave open the possibility that there may be several autonomous affective psychoses.

Until now, the endogenomorphic-cyclothymic axial syndromes have been used in conjunction with the Vienna schizophrenia criteria (Chapter B14). Consequently, literature references for the latter apply here as well.

C11

Taylor/Abrams criteria

Mania

A diagnosis requires all four of the following criteria:

1) Hyperactivity
2) Rapid/pressured speech
3) Euphoric/expansive/irritable mood, with a broad affect
4) No diagnosable coarse brain disease, no psychostimulant drug abuse in the past month, and no medical illness known to cause manic symptoms.

Endogenous depression

The criteria include all three of the following:

1) Sad, dysphoric, or anxious mood
2) Three of a through f:
   a) early morning waking
   b) diurnal mood swing (worse in A.M.)
   c) weight loss of more than five pounds in three weeks
   d) retardation or agitation
   e) suicidal thoughts/behavior
   f) feelings of guilt/hopelessness/worthlessness
3) No diagnosable coarse brain disease, no use of steroids or reserpine in past month, and no medical illness known to cause depressive symptoms.

Sources of criteria: Taylor, M. A. and Abrams, R. (1978) The prevalence of schizophrenia: A reassessment using modern diagnostic criteria. *Am. J. Psychiat.*, **135**:8, 945–8. Taylor, M. A., Redfield, J. and Abrams, R. (1981) Neuropsychological dysfunction in schizophrenia and affective disease. *Biol. Psychiat.*, **16**:5, 467–78.

COMMENTARY

The reasons why Taylor and Abrams established their research instrument have already been described in connection with their criteria for schizophrenia (see Chapter B15). The criteria for mania and endogenous depression published in 1974 (Taylor *et al.* and Abrams *et al.*) are derived from classical descriptions. In particular they refer to *Clinical Psychiatry* by Slater and Roth (1969). They have subsequently been modified into the present formulation (Taylor and Abrams, 1978; Taylor *et al.*, 1981).

The criteria for mania as well as those for endogenous depression contain as an obligatory requirement a certain 'mood.' In this connection it should be mentioned that the Taylor *et al.* (1981) definition of 'mood' differs from that contained in DSM-III, which describes mood as a 'pervasive and sustained emotion' and states that 'mood is to affect as climate is to weather.' In Taylor's opinion, however, 'mood is but a part of an individual's affect, which is a more global function.' Taylor states, moreover, that patients with affective disorders can express a constant mood. Therefore, 'mood' apparently encompasses, according to Taylor, 'emotional resonance.'

The criteria for affective disorders are based mainly on observed or reported symptomatological features. Only the criteria introduced in order to exclude organic or symptomatic psychoses include non-symptomatological anamnestic data.

The criteria for mania contain three obligatory symptomatological elements. Item 3 also accepts the presence of 'irritable mood' and therefore includes states which, in the Vienna criteria, form an independent 'dysphoric' category. The features 'expansive mood' and 'broad affect' have been omitted in the Taylor *et al.* (1981) manual, probably because their definition is not adequately precise. In this book, 'emotional blunting' has been added as an exclusion criterion.

Under item 1 of the criteria for endogenous depression, a 'sad, dysphoric or anxious mood' is included. 'Dysphoric' is not used here in the sense of irritability (which is included in the mania criteria); neither is it employed as in the definition of DSM-III, where it is used as a generic term encompassing anxiety, depression, and irritability. For Taylor and Abrams, 'dysphoric' apparently denotes an affective state which corresponds to the 'depression *sine tristitia*' of classical authors. In his manual, Taylor *et al.* (1981) omits the word 'dysphoric' because of its ambiguity. Under item 2, three out of six criteria are required.

The Taylor/Abrams criteria for affective disorders are essentially empirical. They are additionally oriented upon the endogeny hypothesis which is reflected in the expression 'endogenous depression' (this term is replaced in the Taylor *et al.* manual (1981) by 'major depression').

Indicators for prognosis, time criteria, and elements concerning genetic data are not contained in the instrument. The reasons for this are supposedly identical with those mentioned in connection with the criteria for schizophrenia (see Chapter B15). The presence of the criteria for mania or endogenous depression excludes the diagnosis of schizophrenia, which is a reversal of Jaspers' (1963) hierarchical principle. Consequently, no criteria for schizoaffective disorders have been formulated. The delimitation from reactive psychoses, neuroses, organic psychosyndromes not falling into the category of coarse brain disease, alcoholic states, and personality disorders follow the same lines as already indicated in reference to the schizophrenia criteria (again, see Chapter B15).

The application of the Taylor/Abrams criteria for affective disorders coincides with that described for schizophrenia.

At present the Taylor and Abrams group is working with a modified version of these criteria, which, in addition to schizophrenia, mania, and depression, include a schizoaffective entity. They have not yet been published, because further investigation will be needed to determine their usefulness.

C12

The Newcastle scales (NCS) for the distinction between endogenous and reactive depression

The first Newcastle scale (NCS–1)

Feature	Weight
Adequate personality	+1
No adequate psychogenesis	+2
Distinct quality	+1
Weight loss	+2
Previous episode	+1
Depressive psychomotor activity	+2
Anxiety	−1
Nihilistic delusions	+2
Blames others	−1
Guilt	+1

A score of +6 or more indicates endogenous depression, +5 or less neurotic depression.
Source of criteria: Carney, M. W. P., Roth, M. and Garside, R. F. (1965) The diagnosis of depressive syndromes and the prediction of E.C.T. response. *Brit. J. Psychiat.* **111**, 659–74.

The second Newcastle scale (NCS–2)

Item	Grade	Weight
Sudden onset	Yes	−6
	No	0
Duration	Under 3 months	−6
	3 months – under 1 year	−4
	1 year – under 2 years	−2
	2 years and over	0
Psychological stress	Severe	+12
	Mild/moderate	+6
	None	0
Situational phobias	Marked/incapacitating	+8
	Mild/moderate	+4
	None	0
Persistent depression	Yes	−2
	No	0
Reactivity of depression	Yes	+14
	No	0
Depression worse A.M.	Yes	−16
	No	0
Early waking	Yes	−10
	No	0
Retardation	Yes	−9
	No	0
Delusions	Yes	−7
	No	0

Ranges: −19 and above = Reactive depression; −20 and below = Endogenous depression.
Source of criteria: Roth, M., Gurney, C. and Mountjoy, C. Q. (1983) The Newcastle rating scales. *Acta Psychiat. Scand.*, suppl. **310**, 42–54. This source lacks the item 'Reactivity of depression', amended through a personal communication from Professor Sir Martin Roth; Dr C. Gurney also personally communicated a correct version.

COMMENTARY

Depressive disorders have been traditionally considered to manifest as two distinct entities – endogenous and reactive;* however, this distinction has not gained universal acceptance, and other concepts of the relation-

* In this chapter these two terms are used in lieu of others taken synonymously, such as psychotic and neurotic.

ship between the two entities, such as Kendell's 'psychotic/neurotic continuum' have been advanced (Kendell, 1976). Evidence from research for the traditional dichotomous view increased after the middle of the century (see the review by Kiloh and Garside (1963)). Kiloh and Garside's study, which used factor analysis, provided more support for the nosological distinction between the two entities and constructed a list of their most significant features. The Newcastle scales go a step further. Based on the empirical method for the construction of operational diagnostic criteria (observed by Philipp and Maier in 1987), they are quantified scales for discriminating between the two types of depressive disorders and for predicting outcome of treatment (Roth *et al.*, 1983).

NCS–1, along with a scale for the prediction of ECT response, which will receive no further comment, was elaborated in the following study. Carney *et al.* (1965) selected 35 items, which an earlier study found to be clinically relevant for distinguishing between the two types of depression, as a part of the standard interview of 129 depressive patients admitted to hospital for ECT treatment. The patients were diagnosed as having a definite endogenous, definite neurotic, or doubtful type of depression (relatively few) only after a comprehensive evaluation of all available data. A principal components analysis of the 35 items established the distinction between the two types of depression. The items' weighting coefficients were determined by multiple regression analysis. From the ten items which gave the best diagnostic prediction and their weighting coefficients a diagnostic index was constructed and used to calculate the patients' scores. The distribution obtained was bimodal and also indicated the cut-off point between the two types of depression.

In the original study just reviewed the authors provided definitions for those items which are not self-explanatory. In a later study Carney and Sheffield (1972) expanded the definition for the item 'distinct quality' with the phrase 'patients may even deny depression, despite ample evidence to the contrary, and instead refer to an indescribable mood state' (ibid., p. 36). Eight of the scale's ten items concern endogeny and carry positive weights, the other two concerning reactivity are negatively weighted. The weights of those items applying to a patient are added to determine the score. The cut-off point between the two types of depression is precise: +6 or more is endogenous, +5 or less is reactive. The third, fourth and sixth through tenth items concern cross-sectional symptomatology. The first item appears to be purely longitudinal, yet its definition: 'subjects free from any history of neurotic breakdown and without disabling neurotic symptoms or serious social impairment' (Carney *et al.*, 1965, p. 661) stretches it into cross-sectional evaluation. The fifth item is a longitudinal (previous course) criterion. So is the item 'no adequate psychogenesis,' although its definition requires that it be ongoing to qualify: 'no psychological stress or difficulty continuing to operate after the onset of symptoms and adequate to explain perpetuation of the illness' (Carney *et al.*, 1965, p. 662). 'Depressive psychomotor activity' could be taken simply to be agitation, but its definition includes slowing, up to stupor. The item 'guilt' looks lonely; that feelings alone suffice (Carney *et al.*, 1965) can well be assumed (there is no word 'delusion' as in item 8), but qualification would have been welcome company.

NCS–2 is one of a set of three diagnostic scales published by Gurney (1971) for distinguishing between affective disorders (Roth *et al.*, 1983). Like a decision-tree, according to the result of the anxiety/depression scale, the patient can then be evaluated either by the anxiety scale, the diagnosis being simple anxiety state or agoraphobia, or the depressive scale (NCS–2), the diagnosis being endogenous or reactive depression; if there is no clinical doubt about an anxiety state or depression, the first step may be waived. The scales were developed through an investigation of 149 patients suffering from states of anxiety and depression. The methodology was more complex (including, for instance, two additional principal components analyses for anxiety and depressive items, respectively) than that for the NCS–1 derivation but otherwise essentially similar (compare Carney *et al.*, 1965, with Roth *et al.*, 1972, and Gurney *et al.*, 1972), and the results corroborated the two-type hypothesis (Sandifer *et al.*, 1966).

NCS–2 consists of seven yes/no items and three graded items. In contrast to NCS–1, positive weights correspond to reactivity, negative to endogeny, but the cut-off point is equally precise, between -19 and -20. Seven items, such as two concerning changes in biorhythm, are not shared with NCS–1. The first three items are longitudinal, the rest are cross-sectional criteria. All items are defined (Roth *et al.*, 1972), most are self-explanatory. Psychological stress has a less restrictive definition than in NCS–1 (it is not tied to illness perpetuation), but depressive psychomotor activity is restricted to retardation. The wording of item 6, 'reactivity of depression', is obscure: it resembles what the whole scale is supposed to evaluate, and one may wonder what reactivity refers to – perhaps psychological stress? According to the definition, reactivity is emotional response to positive stimuli. The definition of the item 'delusions' includes mood-incongruent paranoid delusions as well as those of guilt, hypochondriasis, and nihilism. Both scales rule out the possibility that a psychological factor may bring on an endogenous depression. Yet, there is evidence from research that depression cannot be psychopathologically subtyped through the presence or absence of life events (Berner *et al.*, 1983*a*), and Vlissides and Jenner (1982) found no association between NCS–1 stress ratings and ECT treatment outcome for the two types of depression. Because the scales contain no explicit exclusion criteria, Philipp and Maier (1987) observe that they are incompletely operationalized; however, from the original studies (Carney *et al.*, 1965;

Roth *et al.*, 1972) one sees that only patients suffering primarily from depression (and anxiety for the Gurney scales) were selected, and those whose symptoms could be attributable to other causes (organicity, toxicity, non-depressive neuroses, other psychoses) were excluded. Therefore, one can assume that such criteria serve implicity for exclusion.

A number of studies have validated the NCS–1 discrimination between the two types of depression. It was able to predict response to ECT (Vlissides and Jenner, 1982; Roth *et al.*, 1983) and to antidepressant therapy (Carney *et al.*, 1986; Ansseau *et al.*, 1987). Validation has also come from dexamethasone suppression test studies (Coppen *et al.*, 1983; Holden, 1983; Dam *et al.*, 1985; Zimmermann *et al.*, 1986) and other biological findings (Ansseau *et al.*, 1987); a study on clinical, demographic, familial, and psychosocial features of depression (Zimmermann *et al.*, 1987); and a study comparing the sensitivity of four diagnostic criteria for identifying familial recurrent depression (Andreasen *et al.*, 1986). Some authors' studies indicate that a cut-off point of 4 separates the two depressive entities better than 5 (Zimmermann *et al.*, 1986, 1987; Davidson *et al.*, 1984*a*, *b*) and that patients whose scores ranged from 4 to 8 showed the best response to antidepressant therapy (Rao and Coppen, 1979; Abou-Saleh and Coppen, 1983). Establishing a precise cut-off point may be problematical for scales of this nature.

Whenever NCS–2 is evaluated, its older sibling seems to tag along. Several studies found that severity was not measured by NCS–2 or NCS–1 (Carney and Sheffield, 1972; Bech *et al.*, 1980; Carney *et al.*, 1986; Philipp and Maier, 1987); this provides additional support for the binary depression concept. Bech *et al.* (1983) found the average interobserver agreement to be 90% for NCS–1 and 91% for NCS–2. Before using the scales, Bech *et al.* (1980) modified them mainly by introducing intermediate weights into their scoring systems. In this 1980 study the distribution of the NCS–1 scores was unimodal (see also Philipp and Maier, 1987), that of the NCS–2 scores could be characterized only as not normal; however, antidepressant plasma level/effect correlated with the diagnostic dichotomy of both scales. A recent (Bech *et al.*, 1988) antidepressant drug trial proved to be less flattering for both scales: unimodality and no statistically significant differences between classification and treatment response. Katona *et al.* (1987) found that diagnosis according to both scales did not predict response to ECT.

Carney and Sheffield (1972) proposed a 'compromise' hypothesis taking both unitary and binary views of depression into account: reactive depression is a dimension and endogenous depression a category. In support of this distinction, Kendell (1976) found a more solid basis for the endogenous depression concept in the literature. How do the two Newcastle scales fare when compared with other diagnostic criteria for endogenous depression? Philipp and Maier (1987) carried out a study comparing the validity of eight operationalized diagnostic systems – RDC (see Chapter C6); DSM–III (see Chapter C7); MDI (Michigan discrimination index, Feinberg and Carroll, 1982, 1983); both Newcastle scales modified according to Bech *et al.* (1980); TAC (Taylor/Abrams criteria, see Chapter C11); VRC (Vienna research criteria, see Chapter C10); and HES (Hamilton endogenomorphy subscale, Kovacs *et al.*, 1981; Thase *et al.*, 1983) – regarding a random sample of 173 patients with an operationally defined depressive syndrome and, in parallel, those of the sample fulfilling the RDC criteria for major depressive episode. Save for MDI and HES all were valid with respect to homogeneity (construct validity) and with respect to agreement with the ICD–9 (see Chapter C3) diagnosis (concordance validity) in picking up the same latent endogenous depression concept. Of these six systems NCS–2, followed by RDC and NCS–1 and then VRC, showed the highest content and criterion validity with respect to cross-sectional and longitudinal validation criteria. Therefore, Philipp and Maier (1987) concluded that when research into endogenous depression requires an operationalized definition with high validity, the best choice would be one of these four in the order mentioned. Because NCS–2 enjoys the highest restrictivity as well, it is the system of choice for biological investigations, which as a rule require as homogeneous a selection of patients as possible. The Newcastle scales are suitable for investigations where the two types of depression are compared because unequivocal diagnostic attribution is offered. Otherwise, the comparison would be best satisfied by less specific and more sensitive systems such as RDC or VRC that reduce the risk of false positive cases falling to the non-endogenous group. However, the Newcastle scales are not suitable for investigations into the relationship between endogenous depression and the longitudinal items they contain; these items cannot be used for the scales' validation. Philipp and Maier (1987) also question their suitability as scales for the dimensional assessment of endogenous depression because of insufficient Rasch model fitting (Rasch, 1960).

Carney and Sheffield (1972) remark that there are various possibilities for the use of the scales in clinical psychiatry, such as offering quantifying data or helping to decide between endogenous and reactive depression. Roth *et al.* (1983) state: 'Both in relation to clinical practice and scientific research various types of rating and quantified scales can be used with advantage as adjuncts to clinical diagnosis (which has benefitted from the objectivity and stringency of rating scales) rather than as substitutes for it' (ibid., p. 52).

C13

French diagnostic criteria for non specific depressive syndrome

A. At least one of the following:
   1. Depressed mood, characterized by symptoms such as: feeling depressed, sad, blue, hopeless, low.
   2. Loss of interest or pleasure in all or almost all usual activities and pastimes.

B. At least 5 of the following:
   1. Pessimistic attitude toward the future or brooding about past events.
   2. Self-pity.
   3. Anxiety.
   4. Loss of energy, fatigue.
   5. Subjective feelings of restlessness or being slowed down.
   6. Decreased effectiveness or productivity at school, work or home.
   7. Complaints or evidence of diminished ability to think or concentrate.
   8. Poor appetite or significant weight loss (at least 3 kg) when not dieting.
   9. Insomnia or hypersomnia.
   10. Decrease in sexual drive.

C. Criterion A and at least 5 features in criterion B have been present during a period of at least 2 weeks.

D. Not superimposed on chronic schizophrenia, acute delusional psychosis or chronic delusional disorder.

E. Not due to any organic mental disorder.

Source of criteria as well as of diagnostic index in the commentary: Pull, C. B., Pull, M. C. and Pichot, P. (1988) French diagnostic criteria for depression. *Psychiat. and Psychobiol.*, **3**, 321–8.

COMMENTARY

The French empirical diagnostic criteria for non specific depressive syndrome were developed in a way similar to the one chosen to establish the French empirical criteria for non-affective psychoses (see Chapter B16): a representative sample of French psychiatrists was invited to select up to 5 cases of depression corresponding without difficulty to the guidelines of the official French INSERM classification, which is just a nomenclature. The participants were provided with an instrument called LICET-D 100 (Pull *et al.*, 1984) (liste integrée de critères d'evaluation taxonomiques pour depression) assembling all criteria used in the diagnostic systems under investigation and were instructed to evaluate the presence or absence of each of these criteria.

The data gathered from 227 cases were submitted to an univariate statistical analysis. This made it possible to define a basic depressive syndrome, which must be present for French clinicians to make a diagnosis of depression. The syndrome is regarded as provisional, because further statistical evaluation and consideration of the participants' comments and suggestions is necessary, just as it was for the definitive versions of the French empirical criteria for non-affective psychoses.

The INSERM classification splits depression into two major categories: those considered to belong to the manic-depressive psychoses called 'psychotic depression,' whereby the word 'psychotic' is used as a synonym for 'endogenous,' and the 'non-psychotic depressive states.' Not included in these two groups are depressions occurring in schizophrenics, which are regarded as a subtype of chronic schizophrenia and consequently named 'chronic schizophrenia with depression.'

The operational diagnostic tool presented here embraces those criteria for which no significant differences between the group of psychotic depressions and the group of non-psychotic depressions were found; therefore, the authors call it 'criteria for non specific depressive syndrome.'

In the realm of symptomatology the presence of either depressed mood or anhedonia (item A), together with at least five out of ten other symptoms (item B), is required for a period of at least two weeks (item C). The presence of a non-affective psychosis or an organic mental disorder excludes the diagnosis.

The concept of 'non specific depressive syndrome' is quite close to that of 'major depression' in DSM-III (see Chapter C7). As in this system the authors of the French criteria also attempt to reach a further differentiation of this broad group having the identification of an endogenous subgroup in mind. But whereas in DSM-III this purpose is pursued by the formulation of specified criteria for 'major depression with melancholia,' the French have chosen the approach proposed in the first Newcastle scale (see Chapter C12). The criteria for which there was a significant difference between the 'psychotic'* and the 'non-psychotic' depressions were assembled in a list. Twelve criteria were found to be significantly more frequent in the 'psychotic', four in the 'non-psychotic' group. A weight of +1 was attributed to the former, a weight of −1 to the latter, and the index providing the optimal differentiation between the clinical diagnosis of 'psychotic' and 'non-psychotic' was assessed. This led to the following scale, which despite a certain similarity is not composed of the same criteria as the Newcastle scale.

Diagnostic index for psychotic vs non-psychotic depression

1. Distinct quality of depressive mood, i.e. the depressed mood is experienced as being distinctly different from the kind of feelings experienced following the death of a loved one.
2. Lack of reactivity to usually pleasurable stimuli.
3. Social withdrawal.
4. Feelings of inadequacy, loss of self-esteem or self-deprecation.
5. Feelings of worthlessness, self-reproach or excessive or inappropriate guilt.
6. Recurrent thoughts of death, suicidal ideation, wishes to be dead or suicide attempt.
7. Marked psychomotor agitation or retardation.
8. Early morning awakening (at least 2 hours before usual time of awakening).
9. The depression is regularly worse in the morning.
10. Delusions or hallucinations.
11. Previous episodes of 'psychotic' depression.
12. Previous episodes of mania.
13. Tearfulness or crying.
14. Psychosocial stressors (judged to have been significant contributors to the development or exacerbation of the current episode).
15. Superimposed on a personality disorder.
16. Superimposed on a preexisting non-psychotic mental disorder.

Criteria 1 to 12 are given a weight of +1.
Criteria 13 to 16 are given a weight of −1.
Criteria which are absent are scored 0.
A score of 5 or more leads to a diagnosis of psychotic depression.
A score of 4 or less leads to a diagnosis of non-psychotic depression.

* It must be stressed again that 'psychotic depression' in French terminology is not identical with the DSM-III 'psychotic depression' but corresponds to 'major depression with melancholia' in DSM-III.

The diagnostic procedure proposed by Pull *et al.* (1988) thus contains two steps: the first leads to the operational diagnosis of a 'non specific depressive syndrome', the second attempts to decide whether the episode should be considered as endogenous or non-endogenous. This two-step approach presents a considerable advantage compared with the Newcastle scales, which provide no criteria to define a depressive episode and restrict themselves to the differentiation between endogenous and neurotic depressions.

D

SCHIZOAFFECTIVE
PSYCHOSES

The diagnosis and therapy of patients with atypical psychoses has been a subject of research in psychiatry since the end of the last century. In order to differentiate this disorder from schizophrenia and manic-depressive illness, and also to describe new typologies, some authors have focused on its cross-sectional symptomatology, laying special emphasis on such symptoms as mood-incongruent psychotic symptoms (delusions, hallucinations), formal thought disorders, disturbances of affect, and manic or depressive symptoms in general; other authors, meanwhile, have focused on its course (acute onset, full remission, chronic course, etc.).

The term 'schizoaffective' was coined by Kasanin in 1933, and for historical reasons we have included his criteria in our book. In the following years, and up until now, a variety of new descriptions and names have emerged for disorders with a blending of schizophrenic and affective symptomatology, e.g., 'schizophreniform psychosis' (Langfeldt, 1939), 'cycloid psychosis' (Kleist, 1928; Leonhard, 1979; Perris, 1974; Perris and Brockington, 1981), 'remitting schizophrenia' (Vaillant, 1965), 'good prognosis schizophrenia' (Stephens et al., 1966), 'reactive psychosis' (McCabe and Strömgren, 1975), 'psychogenic psychosis' (Faergemann, 1963; Retterstøl, 1978), 'schizophrenieähnliche Emotionspsychosen' (Labhardt, 1963), 'oneiroiden Emotionspsychosen' (Boeters, 1971), 'Legierungspsychosen' (Arnold et al., 1965), 'atypische Psychosen' (Pauleikoff, 1957; Bochnik and Gärtner-Huth, 1982). In addition to Kasanin's criteria, which were formulated by us from his work (Kasanin, 1933) we have included the most well-known and widely used diagnostic criteria for schizoaffective psychoses. These are the research diagnostic criteria (Spitzer et al., 1978b); the criteria for cycloid psychoses (Perris and Brockington, 1981); and the latest version of DSM-III-R (1987). Several authors have formulated specific diagnostic criteria, e.g., Welner et al. (1974); Perris (1974); Kendell (cited in Brockington and Leff, 1979); and Berner et al. (1983a).

The endogenomorphic-schizoaffective axial syndrome (Berner et al.,

1983*a*) does not appear among the criteria, since it is diagnosed in the presence of both the endogenomorphic-cyclothymic axial syndrome (see Chapter C10 on affective disorder) and the endogenomorphic-schizophrenic axial syndrome (see Chapter B14 on schizophrenia).

D1

Kasanin's definition of acute schizoaffective psychoses

CRITERIA

(1) Age 20–30
(2) Usually a history of a previous attack in late adolescence
(3) Normal premorbid personality
(4) Good social and work adjustment
(5) Very sudden onset in a setting of marked emotional turmoil with a distortion of the outside world and presence of false sensory impressions in some cases
(6) Definite and specific environmental stress
(7) Absence of any passivity or withdrawal
(8) Lasts a few weeks or months and followed by recovery

Based on: Kasanin, J. (1933) The acute schizoaffective psychoses *Am. J. Psychiat.* **13**, 97–126.

COMMENTARY

The term 'acute schizoaffective psychoses' was coined by Kasanin (1933) when he described a group of nine cases with a blending of schizophrenic and affective symptoms.

Besides symptomatology (5 and 7), he stressed the importance of precipitating factors (6), premorbid personality (3), social and work adjustment (4), onset and course (2, 5, 8), and age (1). Kasanin formulated his description in his search for homogeneous groups of patients to enhance further research.

Brockington and Leff (1979), however, pointed out that the interrater reliability for the definition listed above was very low.

D2

Perris' criteria for cycloid psychoses

For the criteria of Perris and Brockington (1981) for cycloid psychoses, A to D are necessary:

A. Sudden onset with a rapid change from a state of health to a full blown psychotic condition within a few hours or at most a very few days.

B. Occurrence of at least four of the following symptoms:

   (1) Confusion of some degree, mostly expressed as perplexity or puzzlement.
   (2) Mood incongruent delusions of any kind, most often with a persecutory content.
   (3) Hallucinatory experiences of any kind, often related to themes of death.
   (4) An overwhelming, frightening and pervasive experience of anxiety, not bound to particular situations or circumstances.
   (5) Deep feelings of ecstasy, most often with a religious colouring.
   (6) Motility disturbances of an akinetic or hyperkinetic type which are mostly expressional.
   (7) A particular concern with death.
   (8) Mood swings in the background and not so pronounced as to justify a diagnosis of an affective disorder.

C. Age at onset between 15 and 50 years.
D. Not related to the administration or abuse of any drug or brain injury.

Source of criteria: Perris, C. and Brockington I. F. (1981) Cycloid psychoses and their relation to the major psychoses. In Perris, C., Struwe, G. and Jansson, B. (eds) *Biological Psychiatry*, 447–50. Elsevier: Amsterdam.

COMMENTARY

The diagnostic concept of cycloid psychoses was introduced by Wernicke (1894) with his concept of 'motility psychoses' and developed further by Kleist (1928) with his 'confusional psychoses' and Leonhard (1979) who added the 'anxiety-elation-psychoses.' Perris (1974) published more elaborated criteria, the latest version in 1981 (Perris and Brockington, 1981).

In a study in London, Cutting *et al.* (1978) found that cycloid psychosis could be diagnosed more frequently than mania in their sample of psychotic patients.

The concordance of cycloid psychosis with schizoaffective psychoses (diagnosed by RDC (see Chapter D5) or by Kendell's criteria (Kendell, 1986)) was found to be low in a polydiagnostic study by Brockington *et al.* (1982*b*). Brockington *et al.* (1982*a*) also demonstrated a low concordance between cycloid psychoses and manic-depressive illness. The authors conclude that the diagnosis of cycloid psychosis does not correspond to any of the present Anglo-American diagnostic concepts and think that one-third of the patients with cycloid psychoses could be diagnosed as acute schizophrenics, one-third as schizoaffective disorder manic type, and one-third as depressive with mood-incongruent psychotic symptoms in other concepts.

Validation studies on family history by Perris (1974) revealed a preponderance of cycloid psychoses in psychiatrically ill relatives. Studies on the course of cycloid psychoses by Cutting *et al.* (1978) demonstrated a good prognosis with a high recovery rate (90%) but a high readmission rate (72%). Studies on therapy response by Perris (1974) showed a good response to ECT and lithium prophylaxis.

The criteria of Perris and Brockington consist of:

(1) Symptomatological criteria

   Includes: reported symptons B2, B3, B4, B5, B7, B8; observed symptons A, B1, B6
   Excludes: D

(2) Non-symptomatological criteria

   Includes: onset and duration A; age at onset C

D3

International classification of diseases (ICD), 8th and 9th revisions

295.7 Schizoaffective psychosis

CRITERIA

A psychosis in which pronounced manic or depressive features are intermingled with schizophrenic features and which tends towards remission without permanent defect, but which is prone to recur.

The diagnosis should be made only when both the affective and schizophrenic symptoms are pronounced.

Sources of criteria: ICD 8th Revision (1967) WHO manual of the international statistical classification of diseases V (1965 revision). Geneva: WHO. ICD 9th Revision (1978) Mental disorders: glossary and guide to their classification in accordance with the ninth revision of the international classification of diseases. Geneva: WHO.

COMMENTARY

Since Kraepelin (1919) introduced the dichotomy of dementia praecox and manic-depressive psychosis there has been little agreement on how to deal with cases with a simultaneous or subsequent presence of schizophrenic and manic-depressive syndromes. According to Jaspers' (1963) hierarchical principle these cases were for a long time subsumed mainly under schizophrenia. In ICD-8 and ICD-9 schizoaffective psychoses are incorporated into chapter B5 on schizophrenia.

A weakness of the ICD-concept of schizoaffective psychoses is the restriction on cross-sectional symptomatology which ignores a possible change in syndromatology in consecutive episodes. The majority of patients with schizoaffective psychoses have more than one type of episode in the long-term course (Lenz, 1987; Marneros *et al.*, 1988).

It is well-documented that there can be a longitudinal shift from schizophrenic disorder to affective disorder and vice versa, and that this is not due to wrong diagnosis alone as is frequently proposed (Angst, 1986). However, this is a question that has been neglected by research.

The outcome criteria 'tends towards remission with permanent defect' is very vague and was neglected by authors such as Angst (1986).

Another major problem in the diagnosis of ICD schizoaffective psychoses is the very broad definition of affective symptomatology which makes the use of these diagnostic criteria for research purposes very difficult (Marneros *et al.*, 1981). Of course, the occurrence of depressive (or manic) mood alone is not enough to fulfill the criteria of 'depressive features'. Schizophrenic disorder with depressive or manic mood cannot be differentiated from a schizophrenic disorder without these symptoms on long-term course and outcome (Marneros *et al.*, 1986).

Similarly the vague definition of schizophrenic features would include some mood-incongruent psychotic symptoms, e.g., delusion of persecution based on delusional perception in patients with manic syndrome, including patients with schizoaffective psychosis who would fulfill diagnostic criteria for major affective disorder in DSM-III and DSM-III-R (Lenz, 1987; Berner and Lenz, 1986).

D4

International classification of diseases (ICD), 1989 draft for the 10th revision

Clinical descriptions and diagnostic guidelines

F25 Schizoaffective disorders

These are episodic disorders in which both affective and schizophrenic symptoms are prominent and present within the same episode of illness, preferably simultaneously, but at least within a few days of each other. Their relationship to typical mood disorders (F30–F35) and to schizophrenic disorders (F20–F24) is uncertain. They are given a separate category because they are too common to be ignored. Other conditions in which affective symptoms are superimposed upon or are a part of a pre-existing schizophrenic illness, or in which they co-exist or alternate with other types of persistent delusional disorders, are classified under the appropriate category in F20–F29. Mood-incongruent delusions or hallucinations in affective disorders (F30.21, F31.61, F32.31 or F33.31) do not by themselves justify a diagnosis of schizoaffective disorder.

Patients who suffer from recurrent schizoaffective episodes, particularly those whose symptoms are of the manic type rather than of the depressive type, usually make a full recovery and only rarely develop a defect state.

Diagnostic guidelines

A diagnosis of schizoaffective disorder should only be made when *both* definite schizophrenic and definite affective symptoms are prominent and

Source of criteria: ICD–10 (1989a) *1989 Draft of Chapter V, categories F00–F99 / mental and behavioral disorders. Clinical descriptions and diagnostic guidelines.* April 1989. Division of Mental Health, Geneva: WHO.

present *simultaneously* or within a few days of each other, within the same episode of illness, and when, as a consequence of this, the episode of illness does not meet criteria either for schizophrenia, or for a depressive or manic episode. The term should not be applied to patients who exhibit schizophrenic symptoms and affective symptoms only in different episodes of illness. It is common, for example, for schizophrenics to present with depressive symptoms in the aftermath of a psychotic episode (see post-schizophrenic depression (F20.4)). Some patients have recurrent schizoaffective episodes, which may be either of the manic type or of the depressive type or a mixture of the two. Others have one or two schizoaffective episodes interspersed between typical episodes of mania or depression; in the former case schizoaffective disorder is the appropriate diagnosis. In the latter the occurrence of an occasional schizoaffective episode does not invalidate a diagnosis of bipolar affective disorder or recurrent depressive disorder if the clinical picture is typical in other respects.

F25.0   Schizoaffective disorder, manic type

A disorder in which schizophrenic and manic symptoms are both prominent in the same episode of illness. The abnormality of mood usually takes the form of elation accompanied by increased self-esteem and grandiose ideas, but sometimes excitement or irritability are more obvious and accompanied by aggressive behaviour and persecutory ideas. In both cases there is increased energy, overactivity, impaired concentration, and a loss of normal social inhibition. Delusions of reference, grandeur, or persecution may be present but other more typically schizophrenic symptoms are required to establish the diagnosis. The subject may insist, for example, that his thoughts are being broadcast or interfered with, or that alien forces are trying to control him, or he may report hearing voices of varied kinds or express bizarre delusional ideas that are not merely grandiose or persecutory. Careful questioning is often required to establish that the subject really is experiencing these morbid phenomena, and not merely joking, or talking in metaphors. Schizoaffective disorders, manic type are usually florid psychoses with an acute onset, but although behaviour is often grossly disturbed, full recovery generally occurs within a few weeks.

Diagnostic guidelines

There must be a prominent elevation of mood, or a combination of a less obvious elevation of mood together with increased irritability or excitement. Within the same episode, at least one and preferably two typically schizophrenic symptoms (as specified for schizophrenia (F20), diagnostic guidelines (i)–(iv)) should be clearly present.

This category should be used both for a single schizoaffective episode of the manic type, or for a recurrent disorder in which the majority of episodes are schizoaffective, manic type.

Includes: schizophreniform psychosis, manic type.

F25.1   Schizoaffective disorder, depressive type

A disorder in which schizophrenic and depressive symptoms are both prominent in the same episode of illness. Depression of mood is usually accompanied by several characteristic depressive symptoms or behavioral abnormalities such as retardation, insomnia, loss of energy, appetite or weight, reduction of normal interests, impairment of concentration, guilt, feelings of hopelessness and suicidal thoughts. At the same time or within the same episode other more typically schizophrenic symptoms are present; the subject may insist, for example, that his thoughts are being broadcast or interfered with, or that alien forces are trying to control him. He may be convinced he is being spied upon or plotted against and this is not justified by his own behaviour, or hear voices that are not merely disparaging or condemnatory but talk of killing him or discuss this behaviour between themselves. Schizoaffective episodes of the depressive type are usually less florid and alarming than schizoaffective episodes of the manic type, but they tend to last longer and the prognosis is less favourable. Although the majority recover completely, some eventually develop schizophrenic deterioration.

Diagnostic guidelines

There must be prominent depression, accompanied by at least two characteristic depressive symptoms or associated behavioral abnormalities as listed for depressive episode (F32); within the same episode, at least one and preferably two typically schizophrenic symptoms (as specified for schizophrenia (F20), diagnostic guidelines (i)–(iv)) should be clearly present.

This category should be used for a single schizoaffective episode, depressive type, or for a recurrent disorder in which the majority of episodes are schizoaffective, depressive type.

Includes: schizophreniform psychosis, depressive type.

F25.2   Schizoaffective disorder mixed type

Code here disorders in which schizophrenic symptoms (F20) are co-existent with those of a mixed bipolar affective disorder (F31.6).

Includes: cyclic schizophrenia; mixed schizophrenic and affective psychosis.

F25.8   Other schizoaffective disorders

F25.9   Schizoaffective disorder, unspecified

Includes: schizoaffective psychosis, NOS.

COMMENTARY

Several drafts of ICD–10 were published and, at the time of writing, the final version pending. In Chapter D4 we comment on the April 1989 draft from which the major innovations of ICD–10 can already be seen clearly (see also Chapters B6, C4 and E5).

The April 1989 draft is divided into two parts (ICD–10, April 1989 draft *a, b*): the first contains clinical descriptions and diagnostic guidelines, the second contains operationalized diagnostic criteria for research. The criteria are defined cross-sectionally (and more specifically than in ICD–8 or ICD–9): 'definite schizophrenic and definite affective symptoms present simultaneously or within a few days of each other within the same episode of illness' (ICD–10, 1989*b*, p. 77).

The meaning of these definite symptoms can be seen clearly from the diagnostic criteria for research (ibid.): schizophrenic symptoms are reported or observed symptoms and consist mainly of Schneider's first rank symptoms and Bleuler's basic symptoms (see Chapters B3 and B2).

Affective symptomatology is defined very broadly and it is not easy to differentiate between a patient with schizoaffective disorder, depressive type of moderate severity, and a depressed schizophrenic patient.

The criteria for research are oriented only on the cross-sectional symptomatology, but the diagnostic guidelines are also oriented on the course of the disorder (including different polarity): 'patients who suffer from recurrent schizoaffective episodes, particularly those whose symptoms are of the manic type rather than of the depressive type, usually make a full recovery and only rarely develop a defect state' (ibid., p. 77).

The term schizoaffective should not be applied to patients who exhibit schizophrenic symptoms and affective symptoms in different episodes of the illness and applies only to patients who have recurrent schizoaffective episodes. The 'occurrence of an occasional schizoaffective episode does not invalidate a diagnosis of bipolar affective disorder or recurrent depressive disorder' (ibid., p. 78).

Therefore, the lack of a sufficient longitudinal aspect of diagnosis still seems to be a weakness of ICD–10, although it is well known that the majority of patients with schizoaffective syndromes have more than one type of episode in the long-term course (Angst, 1986; Lenz, 1987; Marneros *et al.*, 1988).

In conclusion it can be said that schizoaffective disorders in ICD–10 (still subsumed under its Chapter F2 on schizophrenia, schizotypal and delusional disorders) are better defined cross-sectionally (despite the difficulty in differentiating from depressed schizophrenia, discussed above) but still are very weakly defined with respect to long-term course. The diagnosis will be easy in patients with recurrent schizoaffective episodes but difficult in patients who additionally have other types of episode. So, from the point of long-term course the concept of schizoaffective disorder seems to be narrower in ICD–10 than in DSM–III–R.

D5

Research diagnostic criteria (RDC)

I. Schizoaffective disorder, manic type

A through E required for the episode of illness being considered.

A. One or more distinct periods with a predominantly elevated, expansive or irritable mood. The elevated, expansive, or irritable mood must be relatively persistent and prominent during some part of the illness or occur frequently. It may alternate with depressive mood. If the disturbance in mood occurs only during periods of alcohol or drug intake or withdrawal from them, it should not be considered here.

B. If mood is elevated or expansive, at least three of the following symptoms must be definitely present to a significant degree, four if mood is only irritable. (For past episodes, because of memory difficulty, one less symptom is required.)

  (1) More active than usual – either socially, at work, at home, sexually, or physically restless.
  (2) More talkative than usual or felt a pressure to keep on talking.
  (3) Flight of ideas (as defined in this manual [Spitzer *et al.*, 1978*b*]) or subjective experience that thoughts are racing.
  (4) Inflated self-esteem (grandiosity, which may be delusional).
  (5) Decreased need for sleep.
  (6) Distractibility, i.e., attention is too easily drawn to unimportant or irrelevant external stimuli.
  (7) Excessive involvement in activities without recognizing the high potential for painful consequences, e.g., buying sprees, sexual indiscretions, foolish business investments, reckless driving.

Source of criteria: Spitzer, R. L., Endicott, J. and Robins, E. (1978*b*) *Research diagnostic criteria (RDC) for a selected group of functional disorders*, third edition. New York State Psychiatric Institute.

C. At least one of the following symptoms suggestive of Schizophrenia is present during the active phase of the illness:

(1) Delusions of being controlled (or influenced) or of thought broadcasting, insertion or withdrawal (as defined in this manual [ibid.]).

(2) Non-affective hallucinations of any type (as defined in this manual [ibid.]) throughout the day for several days or intermittently throughout a one week period.

(3) Auditory hallucinations in which either a voice keeps up a running commentary on the subject's behaviors or thoughts as they occur, or two or more voices converse with each other.

(4) At some time during the period of illness had more than one week when he exhibited *no* prominent depressive or manic symptoms but had delusions or hallucinations.

(5) At some time during the period of illness had more than one week when he exhibited no prominent manic symptoms but had several instances of marked formal thought disorder (as defined in this manual [ibid.]), accompanied by either blunted or inappropriate affect, delusions, or hallucinations of any type, or grossly disorganized behavior.

D. Signs of the illness have lasted at least one week from the onset of a noticeable change in the patient's usual condition (current signs of the illness may not *now* meet Criteria A, B, or C and *may* be residual affective or residual schizophrenic symptoms only, such as mood disturbance, blunted or inappropriate affect, extreme social withdrawal, mild formal thought disorder, or unusual thoughts or perceptual experiences).

E. Affective syndrome overlaps temporally to some degree with an *active* period of schizophrenic-like symptoms (delusions, hallucinations, marked formal thought disorder, bizarre behavior, etc.).

The following qualifying categories should be considered for each subject who currently meets the criteria for Probable or Definite Schizoaffective Disorder, Manic Type.

Subtypes based on the course of the present period of schizoaffective disorder

(1) Acute Schizoaffective Disorder: A through C are required.

A. Sudden onset – less than three months from first signs of increasing psychopathology to any of the core schizophrenic symptoms (criterion C).

B. Short course – continuously ill with significant signs of Schizophrenia for less than three months.

C. Full recovery from any previous episode.

(2) Subacute Schizoaffective Disorder: Course is closer to that of Acute than that of Chronic Schizoaffective Disorder.

> Example: First episode with fairly rapid onset and duration of five months.
> Example: Second episode with onset over a period of six months for this episode and full recovery from first episode.

(3) Subchronic Schizoaffective Disorder: Course is closer to that of Chronic than that of Acute Schizoaffective Disorder.

> Example: Significant signs of Schizophrenia more or less continuously present for at least the past year.
> Example: Second period following a previous period from which he did not fully recover.

(4) Chronic Schizoaffective Disorder: Significant signs of Schizophrenia more or less continuously present for at least the last two years.

Temporal relationship of affective and schizophrenic-like features for current episode

(1) Mainly schizophrenic: Either A or B.

A. Core schizophrenic symptoms listed under **C** in the Schizoaffective criteria were present for at least one week in the absence of manic or depressive features.
B. Prior to the onset of the affective features, subject exhibited the following features which are often associated with Schizophrenia: Social withdrawal, impairment in occupational functioning, eccentric behavior, emotional blunting, or unusual thoughts or perceptual experiences.

(2) Mainly affective: A and B required.

A. Schizophrenic-like symptoms listed under **C** in the Schizoaffective criteria developed simultaneously with or followed manic or depressive symptoms and never were present for a period of at least one week in the absence of the manic or depressive symptoms.
B. Good premorbid social and occupational adjustment.

(3) Other: Does not clearly fit either (1) or (2).

II. Schizoaffective disorder, depressed type

A through **E** are required for the episode of illness being considered.

A. One or more distinct periods with dysphoric mood or pervasive loss of interest or pleasure. The disturbance is characterized by symptoms such as the following: depressed, sad, blue, hopeless, low, down in the dumps, 'don't care anymore', or irritable. The disturbance must be *a major part of the clinical picture* during some part of the illness and relatively persistent or occur frequently. It may not necessarily be the most dominant symptom. It does not include momentary shifts from one dysphoric mood to another dysphoric mood, e.g., anxiety to depression to anger, such as are seen in states of acute psychotic turmoil. If the symptoms in C occur only during periods of alcohol or drug use or withdrawal from them, the diagnosis should be Unspecified Functional Psychosis.

B. At least five of the following symptoms are required for definite and four for probable (for past episodes because of memory difficulty, one less symptom is required).

(1) Poor appetite or weight loss or increased appetite or weight gain (change of one lb. a week over several weeks or ten lbs. a year when not dieting).
(2) Sleep difficulty or sleeping too much.
(3) Loss of energy, fatigability, or tiredness.
(4) Psychomotor retardation or agitation (but not mere subjective feeling of restlessness or being slowed down).
(5) Loss of interest or pleasure in usual activities, including social contact or sex (do not include if limited to a period when delusional or hallucinating). (The loss may not be pervasive.)
(6) Feelings of self-reproach or excessive inappropriate guilt (either may be delusional).
(7) Complaints or evidence of diminished ability to think or concentrate (such as slowed thinking, occupation with delusions or hallucinations).
(8) Recurrent thoughts of death or suicide, or any suicidal behavior.

C. At least one of the following is present:

(1) Delusions of being controlled (or influenced) or of thought broadcasting, insertion, or withdrawal (as defined in this manual [ibid.]).
(2) Non-affective hallucinations of any type (as defined in this manual [ibid.]) throughout the day for several days or intermittently throughout a one week period.
(3) Auditory hallucinations in which either a voice keeps up a running commentary on the subject's behaviors or thoughts as they occur, or two or more voices converse with each other.
(4) At some time during the period of illness had more than one

month when he exhibited no prominent depressive or manic symptoms but had delusions or hallucinations (although typical depressive delusions such as delusions of guilt, sin, poverty, nihilism, or self-deprecation or hallucinations with similar content are not included).

(5) Preoccupation with a delusion or hallucination to the relative exclusion of other symptoms or concerns (other than typical depressive delusions of guilt, sin, poverty, nihilism, or self-deprecation or hallucinations with similar content).

(6) Definite instances of marked formal thought disorder (as defined in this manual [ibid.]) accompanied by either blunted or inappropriate affect, delusions or hallucinations of any type, or grossly disorganized behavior.

D. Signs of the illness have lasted at least one week from the onset of a noticeable change in the patient's usual condition (current signs of the illness may not *now* meet criteria **A**, **B** or **C** and *may* be residual affective or residual schizophrenic symptoms only, such as mood disturbance, blunted or inappropriate affect, extreme social withdrawal, mild formal thought disorder, or unusual thoughts or perceptual experiences.

E. Affective syndrome overlaps temporally to some degree with the active period of schizophrenic-like symptoms (delusions, hallucinations, thought disorder, bizarre behavior).

The following qualifying categories should be considered for each subject who currently meets the criteria for Probable or Definite Schizoaffective Disorder, Depressed Type.

Subtypes based on the course of the present period of Schizoaffective Disorder

(1) Acute Schizoaffective Disorder: A through C are required.

A. Sudden onset – less than three months from first signs of increasing psychopathology to any of the core schizophrenic symptoms (criterion **C**).

B. Short course – continuously ill with significant signs of Schizophrenia for less than three months.

C Full recovery from any previous episode.

(2) Subacute Schizoaffective Disorder: Course is closer to that of Acute than that of Chronic Schizoaffective Disorder.

Example: First episode with fairly rapid onset and duration of five months.

Example: Second episode with onset over a period of six months for this episode and full recovery from first episode.

(3) Subchronic Schizoaffective Disorder: Course is closer to that of Chronic than that of Acute Schizoaffective Disorder.

Example: Significant signs of Schizophrenia more or less continuously present for at least the past year.
Example: Second period following a previous period from which he did not fully recover.

(4) Chronic Schizoaffective Disorder: Significant signs of Schizophrenia more or less continuously present for at least the last two years.

Temporal relationship of affective and schizophrenic-like features for current episode

(1) Mainly schizophrenic: Either A or B.

    A. Core schizophrenic symptoms listed under **C** in the Schizoaffective criteria were present for at least one week in the absence of manic or depressive features.

    B. Prior to the onset of the affective features, subject exhibited the following features which are often associated with Schizophrenia: Social withdrawal, impairment in occupational functioning, eccentric behavior, emotional blunting, or unusual thoughts or perceptual experiences.

(2) Mainly affective: A and B are required.

    A. Schizophrenic-like symptoms listed under **C** in the Schizoaffective criteria developed simultaneously with or followed manic or depressive symptoms and never were present for a period of at least one week in the absence of the manic or depressive symptoms.

    B. Good premorbid social and occupational adjustment.

(3) Other: Does not clearly fit either (1) or (2).

COMMENTARY

The research diagnostic criteria (RDC, Spitzer *et al.*, 1978*b*) were developed as part of a collaborative project on the psychobiology of depressive disorders that was sponsored by the Clinical Research Branch of the National Institute of Mental Health, USA (Maas *et al.*, 1980). They are described as an elaboration, expansion, and modification of the Feighner criteria (Feighner *et al.*, 1972).

In developing the RDC, many additional diagnoses were included, such as schizoaffective disorders and a number of other diagnoses of importance in the differential diagnosis of affective disorders and schizophrenia.

By creating new categories such as schizoaffective disorder, the RDC are able to maintain a narrow definition of disorders such as schizophrenia and still classify most patients. The criteria included in the RDC allow for simultaneous assignment of subjects on the basis of episode diagnosis as well as longitudinal diagnosis, without forcing a decision about which is the most appropriate for a given patient or a given purpose.

Therefore, two diagnoses which are mutually exclusive for the same continuous period of illness (e.g., schizoaffective disorder and manic disorder) may well be appropriate for different episodes.

Schizoaffective disorder, manic type

This category is for subjects who have had an episode of illness that fulfills the criteria for manic syndrome (**A** and **B**) concurrently with at least one of the symptoms suggesting schizophrenia (listed here in **C**). It includes chronic forms even though the term is sometimes limited to acute or episodic psychoses. It also includes forms in which the schizophrenic symptoms are of brief duration compared with the affective symptoms or the converse. The term schizoaffective disorder, rather than schizophrenia, is used to reflect the current uncertainty concerning whether this condition is a subgroup of schizophrenia or more closely related to affective illness. If the symptoms in **C** occur only during periods of alcohol or drug use or withdrawal from them, the diagnosis should be 'other psychiatric disorder.' To a great extent schizoaffective disorder, manic type is a category which helps to 'purify' the samples of schizophrenics and those of affective disorder.

The single items for mania and schizophrenia are discussed in Chapter B8 for RDC schizophrenia and Chapter C6 for RDC affective disorder.

The subtyping of schizoaffective disorder by polarity is of major importance for prognosis and therapy response. Numerous studies reviewed by Clayton (1982), Brockington and Meltzer (1983), and Kendell (1986) have shown that patients with schizoaffective disorder, manic type, closely resemble those with bipolar disorder with regard to family history and therapy response, whereas schizoaffective depressive patients are more heterogeneous in this respect.

The course of the present episode and the temporal relationship of affective and schizophrenic-like features for current episode represent additional guidelines for subtyping schizoaffective disorder. The mainly schizophrenic subtype seems to be associated more frequently with a chronic course (Lenz, 1987) and a poor response to lithium prophylaxis (Mattes and Nayak, 1984).

Schizoaffective disorder, depressed type

This category is for subjects with an episode of illness that fulfills the criteria for a full depressive syndrome (**A** and **B**) but who also have at least one of the symptoms suggesting schizophrenia listed here in **C**. It includes chronic forms even though the term is sometimes limited to acute or episodic psychoses. It also includes forms in which the schizophrenic symptoms are of brief duration compared with the affective symptoms or the converse. The term schizoaffective disorder, rather than schizophrenia, is used to reflect the current uncertainty concerning whether this condition is a subgroup of schizophrenia or more closely related to affective illness.

The single items for depression and schizophrenia are discussed in Chapter B8 for RDC schizophrenia and Chapter C6 for RDC affective disorder.

D6

Diagnostic and statistical manual of mental disorders, third edition (DSM–III)

Schizoaffective disorder 295.70

CRITERIA

The category is retained [see DSM–III, 1980] without diagnostic criteria for those instances in which the clinician is unable to make a differential diagnosis with any degree of certainty between Affective Disorder and either Schizophreniform Disorder or Schizophrenia. Before using the Schizoaffective disorder category, the clinician should consider all of the diagnoses noted in the first paragraph above*, particularly Major Affective Disorders with Psychotic Features.

Examples of cases that may appropriately be diagnosed as Schizoaffective disorder include:

An episode of affective illness in which preoccupation with a mood-incongruent delusion or hallucination dominates the clinical picture when affective symptoms are no longer present.

An episode of illness in which currently there is a full affective syndrome with prominent mood-incongruent psychotic features but in which inadequate information about the presence of previous non-affective psychotic features makes it difficult to differentiate between Schizophrenia or Schizophreniform Disorder (with a superimposed Atypical Affective Disorder) and Affective disorder.

* *Source of criteria: Diagnostic and statistical manual of mental disorders, third edition (DSM–III)* (1980). Washington, DC: American Psychiatric Association.

COMMENTARY

The concept of schizoaffective psychotic illness has for some time meant many things to many different clinicians. In all likelihood, the spectrum of cases called schizoaffective according to these very different clinical concepts is more or less covered in DSM–III by various clinical categories carrying such different names as, for example, schizophreniform disorder, brief psychotic reaction, affective disorder with mood-incongruent psychotic features and so on. The clinical logic with respect to the interrelationships existing between these categories has been considered earlier (see Chapters B9 and B10, and C7 and C8).

In DSM–III, schizoaffective disorder is formally placed in a chapter headed *Psychotic Disorders Not Elsewhere Classified*, the same chapter in which the clinical emphasis in diagnosis is placed on the categories of schizophreniform disorder and brief reactive psychotic disorder (see Chapters B9 and B10). Indeed, not only does DSM–III not explicitly define schizoaffective disorder within the context of this chapter, but the disorder also remains the only diagnostic category without clear-cut diagnostic criteria of its own within DSM–III. In other words, schizoaffective disorder is an ill-defined heterogeneous category, to be used only when one is unable to make a differential diagnosis with any degree of certainty between affective disorder and either schizopheniform disorder or schizophrenia.

D7

Diagnostic and statistical manual of mental disorders, third edition, revised (DSM–III–R)

Schizoaffective disorder 295.70

A. A disturbance during which, at some time, there is either a major depressive or a manic syndrome concurrent with symptoms that meet the A criterion of Schizophrenia. [See Chapter B10]

B. During an episode of the disturbance, there have been delusions or hallucinations for at least two weeks, but no prominent mood symptoms.

C. Schizophrenia has been ruled out, i.e., the duration of all episodes of a mood syndrome has not been brief relative to the total duration of the psychotic disturbance.

D. It cannot be established that an organic factor initiated and maintained the disturbance.

Specify: bipolar type (current or previous manic episode) or depressive type (no current or previous manic episode).

Source of criteria: Diagnostic and statistical manual of mental disorders, third edition, revised (DSM–III–R) (1987). Washington, DC: American Psychiatric Association.

In DSM–III the category of schizoaffective disorder had been retained without diagnostic criteria for those instances in which the clinician is unable to make a differential diagnosis with any degree of certainty between affective disorder and either schizophreniform disorder or schizophrenia.

In DSM–III–R (1987), however, diagnostic criteria for schizoaffective disorder are presented. They consist of symptomatological criteria as inclusion (observed and reported symptoms in A and B) and exclusion criteria (B, C, D), and of non-symptomatological criteria such as the time criterion in B. A bipolar type, moreover, can be differentiated from a depressive type according to current or previous episodes.

Using the DSM–III–R criteria, a diagnosis of schizoaffective disorder can be made when there are schizophrenic symptoms concurrent with an affective syndrome of sufficient duration to exclude schizophrenia and at least two weeks of delusions or hallucinations without prominent mood symptoms. Empirical research, summarized by Clayton (1982), Brockington and Meltzer (1983), and Lenz (1987), has enabled differentiation of schizoaffective disorder by polarity. The criteria can be seen as a further step towards a better descriptive classification of schizoaffective disorder, which can be diagnosed by concurrent and sequential symptomatology.

E

DELUSIONAL (PARANOID) PSYCHOSES

The position of paranoid disorders within the classification of functional psychoses into manic-depressive illness and schizophrenia introduced by Kraepelin is still being disputed. (For this reason we are expanding these comments with some background material). In the 5th edition of his textbook (1896) Kraepelin places the state of dementia paranoides together with dementia praecox and catatonia among the dementing processes and lists the insanity that he came to call paranoia, along with periodical insanity, under the constitutional mental aberrations. In the 6th edition of his textbook (1899) Kraepelin subsequently describes a paranoid form of dementia praecox (divided into two course types) alongside the hebephrenic and catatonic forms and – independently thereof – the clinical picture of paranoia. This precisely expresses the ongoing dilemma concerning the affiliation of paranoid psychoses to schizophrenia: all, part, or none of them.

In like manner a further differentiation appears in the 8th edition (1909–1915), whereby Kraepelin describes the clinical picture of paraphrenia as an entity distinct from both the paranoid form of dementia praecox, subdivided into gravis and mitis types, and paranoia. Dementia paranoides gravis and mitis are characterized by a bizarre and poorly organized delusional symptomatology frequently accompanied by hallucinations, which, after a variable length of time, leads to a variably pronounced demential personality change (mild only in the milder type of course, in which the 'core of the personality' suffers little or no impairment). Paranoia represents a chronic, stable delusional system without any personality change or incoherence. In paraphrenia with its four forms (systematica, expansiva, confabulans, and phantastica) one finds fantastic and bizarre delusional content and hallucinations, but like paranoia no evidence of thought disorder or personality change, even after a long illness course.

Mayer carried out a catamnestic study on 78 paraphrenic patients according to Kraepelinian nomenclature in 1921 and on the basis of the results came to the conclusion that paraphrenia was a form of schizo-phrenia with a mild course, thus disagreeing with the opinion that it constituted a separate entity. Kolle came to the same conclusion about paranoia after an investigation of family histories in 1931. Eugen Bleuler (1911) included the brunt of paranoid illness in his concept of schizo-phrenia, with the exception of typical cases of paranoia and alcohol psychoses.

The concepts presented so far deal exclusively with the question of demarcating paranoid psychoses from schizophrenia. However, as early as 1901, Specht questioned whether certain forms of mood-incongruent delusions might not also arise in the course of affective disorders. The ideas of the Kleist–Leonhard school can be regarded as a continuation of this conception; however, they are dealt with in detail in the section on schizoaffective psychoses (see Part D).

Gaupp (1910) and Kretschmer (1950) emphasize the psychogenetic aspect in the genesis of certain delusional forms. They deserve the credit for having prepared the ground for the present-day multifactorial view concerning the origin of delusional disorders.

Whether paranoid illnesses occurring in advanced age are to be regarded as simply a late manifestation of the disorders already described or as an independent group of illnesses is a further point of discussion.

In Scandinavia Wimmer (1916) developed the concept of the so-called 'psychogenic psychoses.' On the one hand, this led to a restriction of the concept of schizophrenia in that region through the establishment of the obligatory criterion of chronicity (Langfeldt, 1937, 1939). On the other hand, considerable weight was attributed to etio-pathogenetic aspects (reactive paranoid psychosis).

Another particular development, largely independent from the German school, can be found in French psychiatry. In Chapter E1 those chronic and acute delusional states of the French classification for which operational criteria have been established are discussed (Pull *et al.*, 1987*b*).

The diagnostic formulations for paranoid psychoses currently enjoying widespread use arose from the concepts presented heretofore. Part of them were developed within the framework of a comprehensive system of mental disorders (ICD–9, 1978; DSM–III, 1980; DSM–III–R, 1987); the others were created especially in view of an exact classification of non-schizophrenic paranoid disorders (Winokur, 1977; Kendler, 1980*a*).

For the Vienna school, paranoid psychoses occupy a special position regarding classification. It maintains that delusional symptomatology is always a 'superstructure' which may develop on the basis of different morbid processes or may be of purely psychogenic origin. Thus, in contrast to the other classification systems, the bizarreness of delusional content, which is difficult to define operationally, and the presence of certain kinds of hallucinations are not taken as indicators for an underlying schizophrenic process. In the opinion of the Vienna school these individual symptoms constituting a delusion may be classified syndromatologically only as simple delusional syndromes and paraphrenic syndromes (paraphrenia). A definitive nosological diagnosis may be invoked only when the organic origins of the delusional syndrome can be unequivocally established. If this is not the case, a tentative nosological attribution is made to one of the axial syndromes (see Hoche, 1912), which are presented in the corresponding chapters of this book and represent the Vienna research criteria for affective and schizophrenic disorders (see Chapters C10 and B14). Additional information, such as auxiliary organic findings, illness course, genetic data, or response to certain kinds of therapy, may heighten the probability of this tentative cross-sectional diagnosis. In contrast to most of the other diagnostic systems there exists no hierarchical order among the individual axial syndromes.

The latest version of this concept concerning the evaluation of paranoid disorders can be found in Berner *et al.* (1986*a*). A multiaxial classification system is presented therein, whereby axis 1 registers the delusion's structural and constituting elements, axis 2 registers its relationship to reality, and axis 3 registers its content. Axis 4 is reserved to record the axial syndromes if present. Since the delusional symptomatology is regarded as either merely psychogenic or as a superstructure resulting from interactions between a basic organic or endogenous process and individual coping mechanisms and is, therefore, subject to many variations not linked to the illness course, no operational definitions for axes 1–3 are forwarded by the Vienna research criteria.

E1

French empirical diagnostic criteria

French empirical criteria for chronic delusional psychosis (psychose hallucinatoire chronique)

A. At least three of the manifestations 1, 2, 3 or 4 for at least one month

 1) Internal auditory hallucinations
 At least one of the following:

 a) auditory hallucinations in which one or more voices keep up a running commentary on the subject's behavior or thoughts
 b) auditory hallucinations in which one or more voices continuously articulate or echo what the individual is thinking or reading
 c) auditory hallucinations in which two or more voices converse among themselves

 2) Delusional ideas of influence
 At least one of the following:

 a) delusional ideas in which sensations, impulses, or actions are experienced as being imposed by an external force
 b) delusional ideas in which thoughts are experienced as being imposed by an external force (thought insertion)
 c) delusional ideas in which the individual is convinced that he is being robbed of his thoughts (thought withdrawal)
 d) delusional ideas in which the individual is convinced that others know his thoughts (thought broadcasting)

Source of criteria: Pull, C. B., Pull, M. C. and Pichot, P. (1987*b*) Des critères empiriques français pour les psychoses. III. Algorithmes et arbre de décision. *L'Encéphale*, **XIII**, 59–66.

3) Hallucinations of any kind
4) Delusional ideas of any kind

B. Permanent signs of the illness for at least six months with constant presence of at least one of the following:

1) Presence of any one of the manifestations A1, A2, A3 or A4
2) Deterioration from a pre-morbid level of professional, domestic, or educational functioning
3) Deterioration from a pre-morbid level of functioning in social relationships
4) Social isolation or social withdrawal
5) Fantastic, illogical, bizarre, magical or delusion-toned thinking
6) Bizarre or grossly disorganized behavior

C. Does not meet and has never met criterion A1 for chronic schizo-phrenia [see Chapter B16]
D. Does not meet the criteria for acute delusional psychosis [see *bouffée délirante* and Chapter B16, 'acute or subacute delusional episode considered to be schizophrenic']
E. Not due to an organic brain disorder, alcoholism, or drug abuse
F. When an individual meets criteria A and B with the exception of the time proviso of either or both, he is diagnosed as having a 'probable' chronic hallucinatory psychosis
G. Not due to a manic or depressive psychosis

French empirical criteria for chronic interpretative psychoses

A. Delusional ideas for at least one month, characterized by each of the following:

1) Their systematization
   Either a or b:

   a) delusional ideas organized on a single predominating theme
   b) delusional ideas organized on a series of related themes

2) Their theme(s)
   At least one of the following:

   a) delusional ideas of persecution
   b) delusional ideas of jealousy
   c) delusional ideas of grievance (litigious delusion)
   d) erotomanic delusional ideas

3) Their 'mechanism'
   Either a or b:

   a) delusional ideas restricted to delusional ideas of interpretation
   b) delusional ideas of interpretation in the foreground

B. Permanent signs of the illness for at least 6 months with the constant presence of 1 or 2:

    1) Uninterrupted presence of delusional ideas meeting criterion A

    2) Both of the following:

        a) meets the criteria for paranoid personality

        b) deterioration in social relationships since the onset of the illness

C. Does not meet and has never met criterion A1 for chronic schizophrenia (i.e., 'Major disturbance of the train of thought') [see chapter B16]

D. Does not meet the criteria for acute delusional psychosis or chronic hallucinatory psychosis [see chronic delusional psychosis, *bouffée délirante* and Chapter B16, 'acute or subacute delusional episodes considered to be schizophrenic']

E. Not due to an organic brain disorder, alcoholism, or drug abuse

F. When an individual meets criteria A and B with the exception of the time proviso of either or both, he is diagnosed as having a 'probable' chronic interpretative psychosis

G. Not due to a manic or depressive psychosis

French empirical criteria for *bouffée délirante*

A. Delusional ideas characterized by each of the following:

    1) A sudden onset: in less than 48 hours

    2) A multiplicity of themes and delusional 'mechanisms' (polymorphous delusions)

    3) A lack of organization on a single prominent theme or a series of related themes

B. Emotional turmoil without disorientation in time or place, characterized by at least 3 of the following:

    a) sudden changes from one emotional reaction to another, e.g., from anxiety to anger

    b) sudden changes from one dysphoric mood to another; e.g. from euphoria to depression

    c) sudden changes from one type of psychomotor behavior to another, e.g. from agitation to prostration

    d) depersonalization: impairment in perception or awareness of the self and/or derealization: impairment in perception or awareness of the outside world

    e) hallucinations or unusual perceptions of any kind

C. Disappearance of the pathological manifestations in A and B and complete restitution to the pre-morbid state in less than 2 months

D. Absence of any previous psychiatric disorders other than possibly one or more *bouffées délirantes*

E. Not due to an organic brain disorder, alcoholism, or drug abuse

F. Clinical forms:
   Authentic *bouffée délirante* of the Magnan type

   a) meets the criteria for *bouffée délirante*
   b) no obvious stress prior to the onset of the symptoms

   Reactive *bouffée délirante*

   a) meets the criteria for *bouffée délirante*
   b) presence of an obvious stress prior to the onset of the symptoms

G. Not due to a manic or depressive psychosis

COMMENTARY

The special position of the French psychiatric school has already been mentioned in the preliminary comments. Some changes have been made since the first edition of this book through the publication of henceforth operationalized criteria for schizophrenic and delusional psychoses (Pull *et al.*, 1987*b*). The criteria for chronic schizophrenia, aside from a six-month time criterion analogous to DSM–III (see Chapter B9), emphasize disorders of thought and affectivity and largely disregard delusional symptomatology. The criteria for acute or subacute delusional episodes considered to be schizophrenic correspond to the DSM–III concept of schizophreniform disorder and are supposed to take over that part of the earlier French concept of *bouffée délirante* (see Berner *et al.*, 1983*a*) left out of the present one. In addition to these two criteria there exist three groups of non-schizophrenic paranoid psychoses: chronic delusional psychosis (*psychose hallucinatoire chronique*), chronic interpretative psychosis, and *bouffée délirante*.

These operationalized criteria were elaborated through an empirical investigation in the same way as the last version of the French school. After operational definitions were established on the basis of criteria for which the clinicians participating in the study had reached agreement, algorithms were set up and provisional definitions for each of the disorders were published. These were then submitted as a complementary survey to the participants for criticism and suggestions, leading to the final definitions and a decision tree.

The chronic delusional psychosis (*psychose hallucinatoire chronique*) is defined by auditory hallucinations in the form of first rank symptoms, by feelings of being controlled and influenced (delusion of alien control), but also by thought deprivation, which is regarded by the Vienna school as an interpretation of blocking typical for schizophrenic thought disorder. Hallucinations and delusions of any kind also belong to the clinical manifestations. An important criterion is that of chronicity (six months), which also includes a deterioration from a premorbid level of functioning (analogous to the French and DSM–III schizophrenia concepts). Point C of the definition excludes any patient who meets or has ever met the criterion A1 for the chronic schizophrenias. The French schizophrenia concept sets a 40-year age-limit for illness onset but the chronic delusional psychosis concept does not. These latter two facts make it possible to put a large part of the ICD–9 paraphrenia cases into this category, for which too little room remains in DSM–III. Point E excludes organic and exogenous origins. Differential diagnostic problems for the delimitation to manic and depressive psychoses (point G) should hardly ever arise.

The chronic interpretative psychoses represent the French counterpart to the paranoia concept of DSM–III, DSM–III–R, ICD–9, and the 1989 draft for ICD–10 (see Chapters E6, E7, E4 and E5). This group of illnesses could not be diagnosed with the last version of the French empirical diagnostic criteria (see Berner *et al.*, 1983*a*). Persecution, jealousy, grievance, and love constitute the delusional themes. In contrast to DSM–III and DSM–III–R, hallucinations are excluded. Therefore, the French concept closely resembles Kendler's (1980*a*) concept for simple delusional disorder when one disregards the restriction to four delusional themes. Here also the required chronicity is defined by a minimum of six months.

The concept of *bouffée délirante* is derived from cases which would have been attributed to this entity by the earlier version of the French diagnostic criteria through the notion of acute or subacute delusional episodes considered to be schizophrenic (see above). Two types are distinguished: the reactive form triggered by a stress factor and the so-called authentic form (Magnan type). These criteria are comparable with those of the ICD–10 draft's acute delusional episode, but lay more emphasis on the quickly changing affective symptomatology, so that the French *bouffée délirante* notion corresponds more closely to the mixed picture concept of the Hamburg (Kleist, 1928) and Vienna schools (Berner *et al.*, 1986*a*) than does this ICD–10 draft notion. Required also is a *restitutio ad integrum* within two months. The differential diagnostic delimitation to affective psychoses (point G) is essential.

All in all, the latest version of the French empirical diagnostic criteria represents an important further development of the French concept, whose narrow notion of schizophrenia comes closest to that of the Vienna school. An advantage over DSM–III, DSM–III–R, and the 1989 draft for ICD–10 lies in the possibility of adequately diagnosing non-schizophrenic paranoid psychoses, which correspond to the paraphrenia concept of the 8th edition of Kraepelin's textbook (1909–1915).

E2

The Scandinavian concept of reactive paranoid psychoses (Retterstøl)

Paranoid psychoses with marked affective features

The psychoses included in this group are those in which: the affective state is as pronounced as or even more marked than the paranoid symptomatology; the delusions appear relatively comprehensible considering the affective state; the illness has not been associated with symptomatology suggestive of schizophrenia (influence phenomena, autism, ambivalence).

Paranoiac psychoses

The disorders included in this group are those with systematized and firmly knit delusions not subsequently expanding into more fragmented paranoid delusions, and which have not been accompanied by marked affective symptomatology or a symptomatology suggestive of schizophrenia.

Paranoid psychoses without significant affective features

The psychoses included in this group are those in which: the paranoid symptomatology is predominant in relation to the affective; the delusions are not directly comprehensible on the background of the patient's affective state; and the illness has not been accompanied by symptomatology suggestive of schizophrenia or later showed a schizophrenic course.

Source of criteria: Retterstøl, N. (1966) *Paranoid and paranoiac psychoses.* Oslo: Universitetsforlaget.

Paranoid psychoses with schizophreniform symptomatology

In this group are included paranoid reactive psychoses in which the patient on hospitalization also presented symptoms suggestive of schizophrenia with relatively clear consciousness, but where continued observation revealed no further schizophrenic development.

COMMENTARY

Beginning with the twentieth century, Scandinavian psychiatry parted with the German school and followed its own path concerning the classification of paranoid psychoses. Investigations of Birnbaum (1908) and Bonhoeffer (1907), Jaspers' *General psychopathology* (1973; 1st edition 1913), and etio-pathogenetic points of view as central features in the appearance of delusional syndromes, which Kretschmer took into account in his study on the sensitive delusion of reference (1950, 1st edition 1918), formed the basis for this parting. Wimmer (1916) built upon it when he delivered his definition of so-called psychogenic psychoses:

'various clinically independent psychoses, whose main characteristic is that – as a rule in predisposed individuals – they are brought about by mental causes (psychic traumata) in such a way that these traumata are decisive for the moment at which the psychosis begins, for the course it follows (remissions, intermissions, exacerbations), and also frequently for its ceasing. The form and content of the psychosis more or less directly and completely (understandably) reflects the mental causes responsible for its appearance. To these criteria it can also be added that these illnesses show a preponderant tendency towards recovery and especially that they never proceed to dementia' (cited from Retterstøl, 1975, and translated into English by the authors of this book).

The term 'reactive psychosis' was recently agreed upon in all Scandinavian countries. According to Retterstøl these illnesses represent the most frequent diagnosis of psychosis in Norway, especially in initial manifestation, and it is evident that important differences from non-Scandinavian countries concerning psychoses inevitably result. The Scandinavian concept most consistently takes into account the multidimensional view on the origin of mental illnesses brought forth by Kretschmer. A considerable proportion of paranoid psychoses are considered to be 'reactive' in Scandinavia, and if one disregards depressive disorders with mood-congruent delusions, the question of delimitation to schizophrenic psychoses arises as a matter of course. The diagnosis of schizophrenia in Scandinavia is based on Langfeldt (1937). He requires the exclusion of organic illnesses and typical morbid alterations: the 'special type of emotional blunting,' catatonic symptoms, and for paranoid schizophrenics – most important for the delimitation of non-schizophrenic paranoid psychoses – symptoms of depersonalization and derealization in the sense of a serious impairment in ego functioning as well as chronic hallucinations (see Chapter B4). The significant point, however, is that a definitive diagnosis can be established only after a chronic course of at least five years. Here is a criterion of chronicity that, in effect, considerably narrows the diagnosis of schizophrenia; yet, this requirement of a confirmation of diagnosis through course also reflects the problem inherent in the notion of reactivity. After all, Wimmer had already assumed (see above) that reactivity would manifest 'as a rule in predisposed individuals.' Langfeldt (1939) obviated difficulties in differentiating between reactive and schizophrenic psychoses through the concept of schizophreniform psychoses – disorders whose symptoms would indeed raise suspicion of schizophrenia, yet whose further course showed neither the chronicity nor the typical personality changes.

A number of longitudinal studies showed how difficult or often even impossible it is to determine precisely the impact that a psychic trauma may have on different patients or on one and the same patient at different times. They showed, moreover, that the original diagnosis of a reactive paranoid psychosis was in no way connected to cure or episodic course. On the contrary, an initially underestimated proportion of psychoses, as well as those considered to be reactive and devoid of any symptoms suggesting schizophrenia, took on a chronic course and characteristic personality changes. Therefore, transitions take place that are similar to those also described in other disorders, drug-induced psychoses for example. The investigation results of Astrup *et al.* (1962), Astrup and Noreik (1966), Johanson (1964), Noreik *et al.* (1967), and Noreik (1970) showed that a significant proportion of psychoses initially judged to be reactive-paranoid subsequently developed a schizophrenic course. Astrup *et al.* (1962) found a schizophrenic course for as many as 66%; Noreik (1970) found typical schizophrenic personality changes for 36%.

These results led Retterstøl (1975) to the conclusion that 'among the reactive psychoses . . . the paranoid type displays the greater tendency to develop towards schizophrenia' and that 'probably there is a current tendency to over-diagnose this category of psychosis in Scandinavia' (translated into English by the authors of this book).

On the basis of his own investigations Retterstøl (1966, 1970) distinguishes four different forms among the non-schizophrenic reactive paranoid psychoses presented at the outset. The first group consists of paranoid psychoses with pronounced affective features. Retterstøl does not mention whether not only mood-congruent but also mood-incongruent delusional contents are permitted in this form; on the one hand, part of the disorders in this group could be diagnosed with ICD–9 as affective disorders, on the other hand, the classification would most likely be schizoaffective according to ICD–9 (see Chapter B5, 295.7) or affective disorders with mood-incongruent psychotic features according to DSM–III (see Chapter C7, 296.X47). The second group, paranoid psychoses, coincides with the ICD–9 categories (see Chapter E4) 297.0 (simple paranoid state) or 297.1 (paranoia) if one refrains from judging the issue of reactivity. Correspondence to DSM–III (see Chapter E6) is conditional because DSM–III restricts itself to the delusional themes of persecution and jealousy. The third group (paranoid psychoses without pronounced affective features) is related far more to the first category than to the second, because along with the former a stable, systematized, and well-organized delusional structure without tendency to disintegrate is a required criterion. Affective features predominate in the first group, paranoid features in the third.

The fourth group, schizophreniform psychoses according to Retterstøl (1966, see also Langfeldt, 1939), leans on the definition formulated by Langfeldt, because the patient shows autism or ambivalence along with acute onset and triggering factors, yet does not go on to a schizophrenic course. Retterstøl (1966) requires a clear state of consciousness with the onset of symptoms, whereas Langfeldt (1956, 1960) accepts the possibility that a clouded consciousness or isolated affective symptoms may occur also in schizophreniform psychoses and thereby naturally considers the prognosis to be good. These differences further reveal the problems that even authors who are familiar with the nomenclature have with different definitions of clinical pictures. On the basis of the different definitions one can assume that Langfeldt's concept of schizophreniform psychoses is broader than is Retterstøl's; the latter author may well place a part of the former's cases in his third group.

E3

International classification of diseases (ICD), 8th revision

Psychoses (290–299)

Psychosis includes those conditions in which impairment of mental functions has developed to a degree that interferes grossly with insight, ability to meet some of the ordinary demands of life, or adequate contact with reality. It is not an exact or well-defined term. Mental retardation is excluded (310–315).

297 Paranoid states

Includes: a psychosis not classifiable as schizophrenia or affective psychosis, in which delusions, especially of being influenced, persecuted, or treated in some special way, are the main symptoms. The delusions are of a fairly fixed, elaborate, and systematized kind.
Excludes: acute paranoid reaction (298.3); schizophrenia, paranoid type (295.3); alcoholic paranoia (291.3).

297.0 Paranoia

Includes: a rare chronic psychosis in which logically constructed, systematized delusions have developed gradually without concomitant hallucinations or the schizophrenic type of disordered thinking. The delusions are mostly of grandeur (the paranoic prophet or inventor) or somatic abnormality.

Source of criteria: ICD 8th Revision (1967) *WHO manual of the international statistical classification of diseases*, V (1965 revision). Geneva: WHO.

297.1 Involutional paraphrenia

Includes: paranoid psychosis coming on after the age of 45 in which there are conspicuous hallucinations, often in several modalities. Affective symptoms and disordered thinking though present do not dominate the clinical picture, and the personality is well preserved.
Excludes: involutional melancholia (296.0); schizophrenia, paranoid type (295.3).

Inclusion terms

Involutional paranoid state
Late paraphrenia

297.9 Other

Includes: paranoid states that, although in many ways akin to schizophrenia or affective psychosis, cannot readily be classified under any of the preceding categories or as an acute paranoid reaction (298.3).

Inclusion terms

Folie à deux NOS
Paranoid:
   psychosis NOS
   reaction NOS
   state NOS
Sensitiver Beziehungswahn

298 Other psychoses

298.3 Acute paranoid reaction

Includes: mental disorders apparently provoked by some emotional stress that is misconstrued as an attack or threat. Such states are particularly apt to occur in prisoners or as acute reactions to a strange and threatening environment, e.g., in immigrants.

Inclusion terms

Bouffée délirante

298.9 Reactive psychosis unspecified

Inclusion term

Psychogenic psychosis NOS

The chapter on paranoid psychoses in the 8th revision of the ICD, based on the revision of 1965, was published in 1967. At first glance it does not differ appreciably from ICD-9 (1978): yet, some differences are important enough to justify presenting it as a separate chapter.

Compared with the eight possibilities offered by ICD-9 for classifying paranoid psychoses, ICD-8 offers only four. The ICD-9 description of simple paranoid state (297.0) is used in ICD-8 as a general introduction for a rough description of the entire chapter. The description of paranoia (297.0) is taken over nearly word-for-word by ICD-9 (under 297.1). In the ICD-8 version at hand, there is no indication where cases of paranoia querulans are to be classified. It is noteworthy, however, that in the 1971 edition of the German version of ICD-8, but not in the later German-language editions, paranoia querulans does appear as an inclusion term under paranoia (297.0). If this classification of paranoia querulans corresponds to the intention of the ICD-8 authors, then ICD-8 is, in this respect, more logical and consistent than ICD-9, where the entity figures under 297.8 (other paranoid states). Paranoia querulans is, after all, more closely related to 'classical' paranoia than, for example, the *sensitiver Beziehungswahn*, which also appears under 297.8 (see also the corresponding passages in Chapter E4 on ICD-9).

The definition of involutional paraphrenia (297.1) agrees in general with the ICD-9 definition of paraphrenia, save that the former includes an age stipulation (after the age of 45). This restriction obliges the diagnostician, faced with symptoms typical for paraphrenia but beginning in a person 45 or younger with a well-preserved personality, to attribute the psychosis either to paranoid schizophrenia, potentially leading to an unjustified broadening of the schizophrenia concept, or to one of the remaining categories of 297. As for the classification of non-schizophrenic paraphrenic syndromes, ICD-8 is clearly overshadowed by its successor, which realizes the Kraepelinian concept appearing in the text book's 8th edition (1909–1915) to a far greater extent.

Other paranoid states (297.9) represent a residual category whose definition greatly resembles that of ICD-9's 297.8, but whose inclusion terms, aside from the *sensitiver Beziehungswahn*, differ. The position of paranoia querulans has already been dealt with. The other items found under this rubric are paranoid psychosis, reaction, and state NOS, which constitute a separate and more appropriately designated 'unspecified' category (297.9) in ICD-9, and folie à deux, for which ICD-9 (and DSM-III and DSM-III-R as well, see Chapters E6 and E7) also provides a separate category, induced psychosis (297.3).

The Scandinavian influence had only begun to make an impact in time for the 8th revision of the ICD. One does find therein the concept of acute paranoid reaction (298.3), whose definition was taken over nearly word-for-word by ICD-9. And the concept of psychogenic psychosis, which enjoys considerable importance at least for Scandinavian psychiatry, crept into ICD-8 only as a NOS inclusion term under the residual category of reactive psychosis unspecified (298.9).

All in all, with respect to the classification of non-schizophrenic paranoid psychoses, ICD-8 can be regarded as a forerunner of ICD-9, closely associated with the Kraepelinian concept but less thoroughly elaborated.

E4

International classification of diseases (ICD), 9th revision

Psychoses (290–299)

Psychosis includes those conditions in which impairment of mental functions has developed to a degree that interferes grossly with insight, ability to meet some of the ordinary demands of life, or adequate contact with reality. It is not an exact or well-defined term. Mental retardation is excluded (310–315).

297 Paranoid states

Excludes: acute paranoid reaction (298.3)
alcoholic jealousy (291.5)
paranoid schizophrenia (295.3)

297.0 Paranoid state, simple

A psychosis, acute or chronic, not classifiable as schizophrenia or affective psychosis, in which delusions, especially of being influenced, persecuted or treated in some special way, are the main symptoms. The delusions are of a fairly fixed, elaborate and systematized kind.

297.1 Paranoia

A rare chronic psychosis in which logically constructed systematized delusions have developed gradually without concomitant hallucinations

Source of criteria: ICD 9th Revision. (1978) *Mental disorders: glossary and guide to their classification in accordance with the ninth revision of the international classification of diseases.* Geneva: WHO.

or the schizophrenic type of disordered thinking. The delusions are mostly of grandeur (the paranoiac prophet or inventor), persecution or somatic abnormality.

Excludes: paranoid personality disorder (301.0)

297.2 Paraphrenia

Paranoid psychosis in which there are conspicuous hallucinations, often in several modalities. Affective symptoms and disordered thinking, if present, do not dominate the clinical picture and the personality is well-preserved.

Involutional paranoid state
Late paraphrenia

297.3 Induced psychosis

Mainly delusional psychosis, usually chronic and often without florid features, which appears to have developed as a result of a close, if not dependent, relationship with another person who already has an established similar psychosis. The delusions are at least partly shared. The rare cases in which several persons are affected should also be included here.

Folie à deux   Induced paranoid disorder

297.8 Other

Paranoid states which, though in many ways akin to schizophrenic or affective states, cannot readily be classified under any of the preceding rubrics, nor under 298.4.

Paranoia querulans Sensitiver Beziehungswahn
Excludes: senile paranoid state (297.2)

297.9 Unspecified

Paranoid: psychosis NOS
            reaction NOS
            state NOS

298 Other non-organic psychoses

298.3 Acute paranoid reaction

Paranoid states apparently provoked by some emotional stress. The stress is often misconstrued as an attack or threat. Such states are particularly prone to occur in prisoners or as acute reactions to a strange and threatening environment, e.g. in immigrants.

Bouffée délirante
Excludes: paranoid states (297.—)

298.4 Psychogenic paranoid psychosis

Psychogenic or reactive paranoid psychosis of any type which is more protracted than the acute reactions covered in 298.3. Where there is a diagnosis of psychogenic paranoid psychosis which does not specify 'acute' this coding should be made.

Protracted reactive paranoid psychosis

COMMENTARY

General preliminary remarks concerning the origin and dissemination of the international classification of diseases of the WHO (ICD), 9th Revision (1978) can be found in Chapter B5 on schizophrenia.

Among the non-organic paranoid psychoses, six forms of paranoid disorders are listed under the number 297 and two forms under 298. There are no operationalized criteria in a narrower sense for them; nevertheless, two points of view govern the assessment of the clinical pictures described therein:

1. The delimitation from schizophrenic, manic-depressive, and organic illnesses ('exclusion criteria')
2. The symptoms typical for the illnesses ('inclusion criteria')

The exclusion criteria for schizophrenic disorders (paranoid schizophrenia) and organic delusional states (alcoholic jealousy) are mentioned explicitly. Such is not the case for the exclusion of affective disorders. Under simple paranoid state (297.0) one does find a corresponding passage ('not classifiable as . . . affective psychoses'), under paraphrenia (297.2) likewise ('affective symptoms . . ., if present, do not dominate the clinical picture') (ibid.); yet, making a distinction between cases of paraphrenia with pronounced affective features and schizoaffective psychoses (see Chapter B5, 295.7) will often prove to be quite difficult. For the remaining clinical pictures coming under the heading of paranoid psychoses no indication for an exclusion of affective disorders is to be found. Nevertheless, one may gather from the text or the examples cited (for example, induced paranoid disorder, paranoia querulans, *sensitiver Beziehungswahn*) that affective symptoms either do not occur or play at most a subsidiary role. Just how subsidiary is not clear for other paranoid states (297.8); the phrase 'though in many ways akin to . . . affective states' (ibid.) raises the question of their mutual delimitation. Just how this may apply to the entity paranoia querulans included in the concept is also not clear. Even with the broadest interpretation of the Bleulerian schizophrenia concept it is hardly possible to classify paranoia querulans as such on the one hand; on the other hand, the appearance of the hypomanic-sthenic component, not at all obligatory for querulans, should very seldom lead to differential diagnostic difficulties with affective disorders in the narrower sense. Certain problems arise also concerning acute paranoid reactions (298.3) owing to the inclusion of *bouffée délirante* (Magnan, 1893), a concept that is defined in and applied to French criteria. Typical symptoms for this disorder include depression and/or euphoria, whereby a rapid fluctuation of the clinical state within days or hours may occur, so that differential diagnostic difficulties with 'manic-depressive psychosis, other and un-specified' (see Chapter C3, 296.8) may arise. Although 'psychogenic affective psychoses' are explicitly excluded in the latter, one is confronted once again with a differential diagnostic problem.

ICD–9, like DSM–III (1980), belongs to the so-called compromise systems of classification. These combine diagnostic formulations of various psychiatric schools and ways of thinking, which partly contradict and overlap one another, to attain the greatest possible application and dissemination. When one considers that 'reactive psychosis' is the most frequently made diagnosis of a psychotic disorder in Scandinavia (see Retterstøl, 1975), one may fear that the importance attributed to external circumstances and stressful situations which trigger the illness and decisively influence its course will vary enormously in Scandinavia and elsewhere. This problem is apparently insurmountable, the introduction of operationalized criteria notwithstanding.

However, there may be some justification in including induced psycho-sis (297.3) among other non-organic psychoses (298), because it could very well be largely or entirely attributable to a recent life experience. Inci-dentally, the induced psychosis concept also appears in DSM–III, albeit explicitly restricted to the theme of persecution.

As for inclusion criteria, these are essentially determined by certain forms of productive symptomatology (delusions, hallucinations) or by illness course in some cases. Foremost for simple paranoid state (297.0) are 'delusions, especially of being influenced, persecuted or treated in some special way,' for paranoia (297.1) 'delusions . . . mostly of grandeur (the paranoiac prophet or inventor), persecution or somatic abnormality.' The structural elements also carry diagnostic weight for simple paranoid state: 'The delusions are of a fairly fixed, elaborate and systematized kind,' and for paranoia: 'Logically constructed, systematized delusions.'

Paraphrenia (297.2) essentially corresponds to the Kraepelinian concept appearing in the 8th edition of his textbook (1909–1915).

297.9 (unspecified) is reserved as a last possibility for classifying delusional syndromes that find no place under other 297 code number categories because they do not correspond to any of the concepts formula-ted therein.

Differential diagnostic difficulties could possibly arise between the acute paranoid reaction (298.3) and the acute schizophrenic episode (see Chapter B5, 295.4) concepts. Cited in both cases are typical symptoms such as 'a dream-like state with slight clouding of consciousness and perplexity' (295.4) and 'depersonalization/derealization and/or confusion' (in the *bouffées délirantes* included under 298.3). Once again, how much weight should be attributed to triggering factors is an arbitrary decision.

Psychogenic paranoid psychosis (298.4) conforms essentially with the concept of reactive paranoid psychosis according to Scandinavian nomenclature (see Chapter E2).

In summary, the following forms of paranoid disorders are to be diagnosed by means of the criteria cited at the beginning of this section: chronic, stable, and well-systematized delusional syndromes with plausible ('non-bizarre') themes (297.0, 297.1, 297.8); a variety of psychoses whose rich, productive symptomatology does not exclude bizarre themes, yet in whose courses deficiency states do not develop (297.2, including late-onset paranoid disorders); induced psychoses (297.3) free of thematic restrictions; and acute (298.3) or longer-lasting (298.4) paranoid psychoses for which external events precipitate onset and determine illness course.

E5

International classification of diseases (ICD), 1989 draft for the 10th revision

F22 Persistent delusional disorders

This group includes a variety of disorders in which longstanding delusions constitute the only, or the most conspicuous, clinical characteristic and which cannot be classified as organic, schizophrenic or affective. They are probably heterogeneous but appear to be unrelated to schizophrenia. The relative importance of genetic factors, personality characteristics and life circumstances in their genesis is uncertain, and probably variable.

F22.0 Delusional disorder

A rather ill defined disorder characterized by the development either of a single delusion or of a set of related delusions which are usually persistent and sometimes lifelong. The content of the delusion or delusions is very variable. Often they are persecutory, hypochondriacal, or grandiose but they may be concerned with litigation or jealousy, or express a conviction that the subject's body is misshapen, or that others think that he smells or is homosexual. Other psychopathology is characteristically absent but depressive symptoms may be present intermittently and olfactory and tactile hallucinations may develop in some cases. Clear and persistent auditory hallucinations (voices), schizophrenia symptoms such as delusions of control and marked blunting of affect, and definite evidence of brain disease are all incompatible with this diagnosis. However, particularly in elderly patients, the presence of occasional or transitory

Source of criteria: ICD–10 (1989a) 1989 Draft of chapter V, categories F00–F99/mental and behavioral disorders. Clinical descriptions and diagnostic guidelines. April 1989. Division of Mental Health, Geneva: WHO.

auditory hallucinations does not rule out this diagnosis, so long as they are not typically schizophrenic and form only a small part of the overall clinical picture. The onset is commonly in middle age but sometimes, particularly in the case of beliefs about having a misshapen body, it is in early adult life. The content of the delusion, and the timing of its emergence, can often be related to the subject's life situation, e.g. persecutory delusions in members of minorities. Apart from actions and attitudes directly related to the delusion or delusional system, affect, speech and behaviour are normal.

Diagnostic guidelines

Delusions constitute the only or most conspicuous clinical characteristic. The delusion or delusions must be present for at least three months and be clearly personal rather than subcultural. Depressive symptoms or even a full blown depressive episode (F32) may be present intermittently, provided the delusion persists at times when there is no disturbance of mood. There must be no evidence of brain disease, no or only occasional auditory hallucinations, and no history of schizophrenic symptoms (delusions of control, thought broadcasting etc.)

Includes: late paraphrenia; paranoia; paranoid state; paranoid psychosis NOS.

F22.8 Other persistent delusional disorders

This is a residual category for persistent delusional disorders which do not meet criteria for delusional disorder (F22.0). Code here disorders in which the delusion or delusions are accompanied by persistent hallucinatory voices or by schizophrenic symptoms which are insufficient to meet criteria for schizophrenia (F20). Delusional disorders which have lasted for less than three months should, however, be coded, at least temporarily, under F23.

Includes: involutional paranoid state; paranoia querulans; sensitiver Beziehungswahn.

F22.9 Persistent delusional disorder, unspecified

F23 Acute and transient psychotic disorders

Introduction

Systematic clinical information that would provide definitive guidance on the classification of acute psychotic disorders is not yet available, and the limited data and clinical tradition that therefore must be used instead do not give rise to concepts that can be clearly defined and separated from each other. In the absence of a tried and tested multi-axial system, the method used here to avoid diagnostic confusion is to construct a diagnostic sequence which reflects the order of priority given to selected key features of the disorder. The order of priority used here is:

(i) an acute onset (within two weeks), as the defining feature of the whole group
(ii) the presence of typical syndromes
(iii) the presence of associated acute stress.

The classification is nevertheless arranged so that those who do not agree with this order of priority can still identify acute psychotic disorders with each of these specified features. In addition, it is recommended that whenever possible a further sub-division of onset be used, if applicable, of abrupt onset (within 48 hours) for all the disorders of this group.

Acute onset is defined as a change from a state without psychotic features to a clearly abnormal psychotic state, within a period of two weeks or less. There is some evidence that acute onset is associated with a good outcome, and it may be that the more abrupt the onset, the better the outcome. It is therefore recommended that, whenever appropriate, an abrupt onset be specified, *abrupt* being defined as a change, as for acute above, but within a period of 48 hours or less.

The *typical syndromes* that have been selected are, first, the rapidly changing and variable state, called here 'polymorphic', that has been given prominence in acute psychotic states by authorities in several different countries, and second, the presence of typical schizophrenic symptoms.

Associated acute stress has also been specified, in view of its traditional linkage with acute psychosis. The limited evidence available, however, indicates that a substantial proportion of acute psychotic disorders arise without associated stress, so provision has been made for the presence or absence of stress to be recorded. Associated acute stress is taken to mean that the first psychotic symptoms occurred within about two weeks of one or more events that would be regarded as stressful to most persons under similar circumstances in the culture of the person concerned. Typical events would be bereavements, unexpected loss of partners or jobs, marriage, or the psychological trauma of combat, terrorism and torture. Long-standing difficulties or problems should not be included as a source of stress in this context.

Complete recovery usually occurs within two to three months, often within a few weeks or even days, and only a small proportion of patients with these disorders develop persistent and disabling states. Unfortunately the present state of knowledge does not allow the early prediction of that small proportion of patients who will not have a rapid recovery.

These clinical descriptions and diagnostic guidelines are written on the assumption that they will be used by clinicians who may need to make a diagnosis when having to assess and treat patients within a few days or weeks of the onset of the disorder, not knowing how long the disorder will last. A number of reminders about the time limits and transition from one disorder to another have therefore been included, so as to alert those recording the diagnosis to the need to keep them up to date.

The nomenclature of these acute disorders is as uncertain as their nosological status, but an attempt has been made to use simple and familiar terms. Psychotic disorder is used as a term of convenience for all the members of this group (psychotic is defined in the general intro-duction, [ICD–10, 1989 draft] page 4) with an additional qualifying term indicating the major defining feature of each separate type as it takes its turn in the sequence noted above.

Diagnostic guidelines

None of the disorders in the group satisfy the criteria for either manic (F30) or depressive (F32) episodes, although emotional changes and individual affective symptoms may be prominent from time to time.

These disorders are also defined by the absence of organic causation, such as states of concussion, deliria or dementia. Perplexity, preoccu-pation and inattention to the immediate conversation are often present but if they are so marked or persistent as to suggest delirium or dementia of organic cause, the diagnosis should be delayed until investigation or observation has clarified this point. Similarly, disorders in F23 should not be diagnosed in the presence of obvious intoxication by drugs or alcohol. However, the recent occurrence of a minor increase in the consumption of, for instance, alcohol or marijuana, with no evidence of severe intoxication or disorientation, should not rule out the diagnosis of one of these acute psychotic disorders.

An important point about both the 48 hour and the two week criteria is that these are not put forward as the times of maximum severity and disturbance, but as times by which the psychotic symptoms are obvious, and disruptive of at least some aspects of daily life and work. The peak disturbance may be reached later in both instances; the symptoms and disturbance only have to be obvious by the stated times, and usually in the sense that they will have brought the subject into contact with some form of helping or medical agency. Prodromal periods of anxiety, depression, social withdrawal or mildly abnormal behaviour do not qualify for inclusion in these periods of time.

A fifth character may be used to indicate whether or not the acute psychotic disorder is associated with acute stress:

F23.x0   without associated acute stress
F23.x1   with associated acute stress

Includes: acute (undifferentiated) schizophrenia; *bouffée délirante*; cycloid psychosis; oneirophrenia; paranoid reaction; psychogenic (paranoid) psychosis; reactive psychosis; schizophrenic reaction; schizo-phreniform attack or psychosis.

F23.0 Acute polymorphic psychotic disorder (without symptoms of schizophrenia)

An acute psychotic disorder in which hallucinations, delusions, and perceptual disturbances are obvious, but are markedly variable and changing from day to day or even from hour to hour. Emotional turmoil with intense transient feelings of happiness and ecstasy or anxieties and irritability, are also frequently present. This polymorphic and unstable changing clinical picture is characteristic, and even though individual affective or psychotic symptoms may at times be prominent, the criteria for manic episode (F30), depressive episode (F32) or schizophrenia (F20) are not fulfilled. This disorder is particularly likely to have an abrupt onset (within 48 hours) and a rapid resolution of symptoms; in a large propor-tion there is no obvious precipitating stress.

If the symptoms persist for more than three months, the diagnosis should be changed. (Persistent delusional disorder (F22) or other non-organic psychotic disorder (F28) are likely to be the most appropriate.)

Diagnostic guidelines

For a definite diagnosis (i) the onset must be acute (from a non-psychotic state to a clearly psychotic state within two weeks or less); (ii) there must be several types of hallucinations or delusions, changing in both type and intensity from day to day or within the same day; (iii) there should be a similarly varying emotional state, and (iv) in spite of the variety of symptoms, none should be present with sufficient consistency to fulfil the criteria for schizophrenia (F20) or for manic or depressive episode (F30 or F32).

F23.1 Acute polymorphic psychotic disorder with symptoms of schizophrenia

An acute psychotic disorder which meets the descriptive criteria for acute polymorphic psychotic disorder (F23.0) and in which in addition typically schizophrenic symptoms (F20) are consistently present.

Diagnostic guidelines

For a definite diagnosis (i) the criteria (i), (ii), and (iii), specified for acute polymorphic psychotic disorder (F23.0) must be fulfilled, and (ii) in addition, symptoms that fulfil the criteria for schizophrenia (F20) must have been present for the majority of the time since an obviously clinical picture has been established.

If the schizophrenic symptoms persist for more than one month, the diagnosis should be changed to schizophrenia (F20).

F23.2 Acute schizophrenia-like psychotic disorder

An acute psychotic disorder in which the psychotic symptoms are comparatively stable and fulfil the criteria for schizophrenia (F20), but which have lasted for less than one month. Some degree of emotional variability or instability may be present, but not to the extent described in acute polymorphic psychotic disorder (F23.0).

Diagnostic guidelines

For a definite diagnosis (i) the onset of psychotic symptoms must be acute (two weeks or less from a non-psychotic to a clearly psychotic state); (ii) symptoms that fulfil the criteria for schizophrenia (F20) must have been present for the majority of the time since an obviously psychotic clinical picture has been established; (iii) the criteria for acute polymorphic psychotic disorder are not fulfilled.

If the schizophrenic symptoms last for more than one month, the diagnosis should be changed to schizophrenia (F20).

F23.3 Other acute predominantly delusional psychotic disorder

An acute psychotic disorder in which comparatively stable delusions or hallucinations are the main clinical features, but they do not fulfil the criteria for schizophrenia (F20). Delusions of persecution or reference are common, and hallucinations are usually auditory (voices talking directly to the patient).

Diagnostic guidelines

For a definite diagnosis (i) the onset of psychotic symptoms must be acute (two weeks or less from a non-psychotic to a clearly psychotic state); (ii) delusions or hallucinations must have been present for the majority of the time since an obviously psychotic state has been established; and (iii) the criteria for neither schizophrenia (F20) nor acute polymorphic psychotic disorder (F23.0) are fulfilled.

If delusions persist for more than three months, the diagnosis should be changed to persistent delusional disorder (F22). If only hallucinations persist for more than three months, the diagnosis should be changed to other non-organic psychotic disorder (F28).

F23.8 Other acute and transient psychotic disorders

Code here any other acute psychotic disorders which are unclassifiable under any other disorders in F23 (such as acute psychotic states in which definite delusions or hallucinations occur, but persist for only small proportions of the time). States of undifferentiated excitement should also be coded here if more information about the details of the patient's mental state is not available, so long as there is evidence that an organic cause is not present.

F23.9 Acute and transient psychotic disorder, unspecified

F24 Induced delusional disorder (folie à deux)

A rare delusional disorder shared by two persons with close emotional links. Only one of the pair suffers from a genuine psychotic disorder; the delusions are induced in the other and are usually given up when the two are separated. The psychotic illness of the dominant member is most commonly schizophrenic but this is not necessarily or invariably so. Both the original delusions in the dominant member and their induced counterpart are usually chronic and either persecutory or grandiose in nature. Occasionally the condition may involve more than two people. Delusional beliefs are only transmitted this way under uncommon circumstances. Almost invariably the two people concerned have an unusually close relationship and are isolated, by language, culture or geography, from others. The individual in whom the delusions are induced is usually also dependent on or subservient to the partner with the genuine psychosis.

Diagnostic guidelines

A diagnosis of induced delusional disorder should only be made if: (i) two people share the same delusion or delusional system and support one another in this belief; (ii) they have an unusually close relationship of the kind described above; (iii) there is temporal or other contextual evidence that the delusion was induced in the passive member of the pair by contact with the active partner. Induced hallucinations are unusual but do not negate the diagnosis. However, if there are reasons for believing that two people living together have independent psychotic disorders neither should be coded here, even if some of their delusions are shared.

Includes: induced paranoid disorder.
Excludes: folie simultanée.

F28 Other non-organic psychotic disorders

Classify here: (i) Psychotic disorders which do not meet the criteria for schizophrenia (F20) or for psychotic types of mood (affective) disorders (F3); and (ii) psychotic disorders which do not meet the symptomatic criteria for persistent delusional disorders (F22).

Includes: chronic hallucinatory psychosis NOS.

F29 Non-organic psychosis, unspecified

To be used only as a last resort, when no other term can be used. For mental disorder, unspecified, use F99.

Includes: psychosis NOS.
Excludes: mental disorder NOS (F99); organic or symptomatic psychosis NOS (F09).

The April 1989 draft for the 10th revision of the ICD differs from ICD–9
(1978) in some important ways with respect to the classification of
endogenous psychoses. A dichotomous subclassification exists for these
disorders, whereby it is noteworthy that in the first draft versions the
schizoaffective category was classified among the affective psychoses, but
in the last version it reappeared among schizophrenia, schizotypal states,
and delusional disorders (F2). Under this heading appear, next to the
schizophrenias and schizotypal states, the groups of persistent delusional
disorders (F22), acute and transient psychotic disorders (F23), induced
delusional disorder (F24), and the two residual categories for cases not
classifiable elsewhere (F28, F29) to be discussed in this chapter. In
addition to the general descriptions, diagnostic guidelines are offered for
all but the residual categories. These guidelines nearly always define the
corresponding morbid states better and more clearly than do the exem-
plary descriptions in the ICD–9. In April 1989 a first version of diagnostic
criteria for research (ICD–10, 1989b) was published together with the
diagnostic guidelines (ICD–10, 1989a). These research criteria will be
mentioned at the end of this chapter.

The ICD–10 draft definition of schizophrenia (see Chapter B6) establishes the boundary between this disorder and the various paranoid
psychoses.

Persistent delusional disorder comprises three subgroups: delusional
disorder (paranoia) (F22.0), the residual category of other persistent
delusional disorders (F22.8), and, as a last possibility, persistent delusional disorder, unspecified (F22.9). For paranoia, the ICD–10 draft offers
more examples of delusional themes, such as litigation and jealousy, than
just the three (persecutory, hypochondriacal, grandiose) of its pre-
decessor, following a similar trend set by DSM–III–R with respect to
DSM–III (see Chapters E7 and E6). The presence of auditory hallucinations defined as voices exclude the diagnosis when 'clear and persistent;' when, however, the transitory voices diagnostically compatible with
paranoia (the guidelines qualify them as 'occasional') are not schizophrenic but do seem to be clinically significant, the diagnostician can
always fall back on the F22.8 category. Olfactory and tactile hallucinations, on the other hand, may occur to any extent whatever; all other

hallucinations are excluded. The chronicity of the illness is clearly indicated in the description; the diagnostic guidelines specify a minimal duration of three months. With respect to the possibility of the manifestation of depressive symptoms during paranoia, an important distinction exists between the ICD–10 draft on the one hand and the DSM–III and Kendler criteria (1980a) on the other: the latter stipulate that affective symptoms be either absent while the patient is delusional or relatively short-lived compared with the delusional symptoms; the ICD–10 draft stipulates that the delusional symptoms persist during the absence and during the presence of depressive symptoms 'or even a full blown depressive episode' which may intermittently occur. That 'late paraphrenia' is included in delusional disorder (F22.0) represents a partial departure from the Kraepelinian concept. Aside from the residual category 'persistent delusional disorder, unspecified' (F22.9), the possibility still remains for non-schizophrenic, chronic delusional syndromes with atypical symptomatology (for instance, 'accompanied by persistent hallucinatory voices or by schizophrenic symptoms which are insufficient to meet criteria for schizophrenia') to be classified under 'other persistent delusional disorders' (F22.8). It is not entirely clear why cases of paranoia querulans also fall under this rubric (see Chapter E4). Even less clear is the inclusion of *sensitiver Beziehungswahn* here because it seems to fulfill the criteria for paranoia listed under F22.0 (the delusional content is 'very variable' and may, for example, 'express a conviction that the subject's body is misshapen or that others think that he smells or is homosexual.').

In contrast to the relatively uniform category described, acute and transient psychotic disorders (F23) represents an attempt to group polymorphic acute psychotic states together through the acuteness and transitoriness that they all share. Since a more prolonged illness course cannot be predicted at onset, the possibility of a subsequent diagnostic reattribution (above all to schizophrenia or persistent delusional disorders) is left open. The three most important features of the category as a whole are listed according to priority, the most important one being acute onset (within two weeks). The third one, the presence of associated acute stress, is optional; this feature's presence or absence may be recorded by a fifth character. The second one concerns the presence of typical syndromes: the rapidly changing, variable 'polymorphic' state and typical schizophrenic symptoms. Although 'complete recovery usually occurs within two to three months,' the two subcategory disorders with schizophrenic symptoms (F23.1 and F23.2) set a one-month limit. Unmistakable manic-depressive illness and organicity are exclusion criteria, but allowance is given to less important affective disturbances and recent increase of alcohol- or drug-intake which was insufficient to provoke organic symptoms. The number of illness entities qualifying for inclusion is generous, ranging from acute schizophrenia over *bouffée délirante* and cycloid psychosis to paranoid reaction, psychogenic (paranoid) psychosis, and schizophreniform psychosis.

Acute polymorphic psychotic disorder (F23.0) is a state in which hallucinations, delusions, affective symptoms, and emotional turmoil are unmistakable and unstable, not only changing as rapidly as 'from hour to hour' in nature but also giving way to one another in prominence. The picture is quite reminiscent of the French *bouffée délirante* (see Chapter E1 on the French criteria in this section).

An illness duration exceeding three months should lead to diagnostic reattribution, the most likely candidates being persistent delusional disorder (F22) or other non-organic psychotic disorder (F28).

The distinction between acute polymorphic psychotic disorder with symptoms of schizophrenia (F23.1) and acute schizophrenia-like psychotic disorder (F23.2) will, in most cases, have to be abitrary. The time criterion (less than one month) is identical, schizophrenic symptoms must be present in both for the majority of time, and diagnoses have to be changed to schizophrenia, if symptoms persist for more than one month. The only difference is that in F23.1 the criteria for acute polymorphic psychotic disorder (F23.0) have to be fulfilled whereas F23.2 should describe 'comparatively stable' clinical pictures, where 'some degree of emotional variability or instability may be present, but not to the extent described in acute polymorphic psychotic disorder.'

To be classified under other acute predominantly delusional psychotic disorders (F23.3) are states which, in contrast to the previous acute categories, are characterized by relatively stable delusions or hallucinations and do not satisfy the criteria for schizophrenia or acute polymorphic psychotic disorder. This is also the category under which cases that correspond to the ICD–9 paraphrenia definition, but seldom begin acutely, would be ordered, at least up until a change of diagnosis after three months to other non-organic psychotic disorders (F28) or persistent delusional disorders (F22).

Other acute and transient psychotic disorders (F23.8) and unspecified acute and transient psychotic disorder (F23.9) represent two residual categories.

As in ICD–9 and in DSM–III and DSM–III–R there exists also in the ICD–10 draft the concept of induced delusional disorder, or *folie à deux* (F24).

Save for the residual category non-organic psychosis, unspecified (F29), other non-organic psychotic disorders (F28) represents a wholly negatively defined category (through the exclusion of schizophrenic, manic-depressive, and persistent delusional disorders), whose existence should call forth fundamental reflexion. (Chronic hallucinatory psychosis NOS is offered as a typical example for it). The various categories of schizophrenia, delusional disorder, schizoaffective disorder, etc., should really suffice to classify the vast majority of all illnesses which could come into consideration. If one examines the definition of schizophrenia which is, after all, narrower than that of ICD–9, the suspicion already arises that perhaps too little room is left for longer lasting as opposed to acute paranoid-hallucinatory syndromes (F23, acute and transient psychotic disorders, seems to carry a disproportionate number of subcategories compared with the other categories). This can either prompt the diagnostician to apply the diagnosis of schizophrenia very generously, which surely does not correspond to the intention of this more narrowly conceived definition, or oblige him to choose a residual category (such as F28, other non-organic psychotic disorders), which ought to be reserved only for unclear cases, when he is confronted with cases – even well-documented ones – that evade diagnostic attribution according to the system at hand.

The Diagnostic Criteria for Research (ICD–10, 1989*b*) should provide – according to its introduction – a greater degree of detail and precision compared with the Diagnostic Guidelines, reflecting the modern trend in psychiatric diagnosis. However, the version available until completion of the manuscript can be seen only as a first step in this direction. If the guidelines are taken together with the research criteria, a number of inconsistencies and confusing formulations appear. There is still a need for a fuller version in the future.

E6

Diagnostic and statistical manual of mental disorders, third edition (DSM–III)

CRITERIA

Diagnostic criteria for paranoid disorder

A. Persistent persecutory delusions or delusional jealousy.
B. Emotion and behavior appropriate to the content of the delusional system.
C. Duration of illness of at least one week.
D. None of the symptoms of criterion A of Schizophrenia [DSM–III, p. 188], such as bizarre delusions, incoherence, or marked loosening of associations.
E. No prominent hallucinations.
F. The full depressive or manic syndrome (criteria A and B of major depressive or manic episode [ibid.], p. 213, and p. 208) is either not present, developed after any psychotic symptoms, or was brief in duration relative to the duration of the psychotic symptoms.
G. Not due to an Organic Mental Disorder.

297.10 Paranoia

The essential feature is the insidious development of a Paranoid Disorder with a permanent and unshakable delusional system accompanied by preservation of clear and orderly thinking. Frequently the individual considers himself or herself endowed with unique and superior abilities. Chronic forms of 'conjugal paranoia' and Involutional Paranoid State should be classified here.

Source of criteria: Diagnostic and statistical manual of mental disorders, third edition (DSM–III) (1980). Washington, DC: American Psychiatric Association.

Diagnostic criteria for paranoia
  A. Meets the criteria for Paranoid Disorder ([ibid.] p. 196).
  B. A chronic and stable persecutory delusional system of at least six months' duration.
  C. Does not meet the criteria for Shared Paranoid Disorder.

297.30 Shared paranoid disorder

The essential feature is a persecutory delusional system that develops as a result of a close relationship with another person who already has a disorder with persecutory delusions. The delusions are at least partly shared. Usually, if the relationship with the other person is interrupted, the delusional beliefs will diminish or disappear. In the past this disorder has been termed Folie à deux, although in rare cases, more than two persons may be involved.

Diagnostic criteria for shared paranoid disorder
  A. Meets the criteria for Paranoid Disorder ([ibid.] p. 196).
  B. Delusional system develops as a result of a close relationship with another person or persons who have an established disorder with persecutory delusions.

298.30 Acute paranoid disorder

The essential feature is a Paranoid Disorder of less than six months' duration. It is most commonly seen in individuals who have experienced drastic changes in their environment, such as immigrants, refugees, prisoners of war, inductees into military services, or people leaving home for the first time. The onset is usually relatively sudden and the condition rarely becomes chronic.

Diagnostic criteria for acute paranoid disorder
  A. Meets the criteria for Paranoid Disorder ([ibid.] p. 196).
  B. Duration of less than six months.
  C. Does not meet the criteria for Shared Paranoid Disorder ([ibid.] p. 197).

297.90 Atypical paranoid disorder

This is a residual category for Paranoid Disorders not classifiable above.

298.90 Atypical psychosis

This is a residual category for cases in which there are psychotic symptoms (delusions, hallucinations, incoherence, loosening of associations, markedly illogical thinking, or behavior that is grossly disorganized or catatonic) that do not meet the criteria for any specific mental disorder.
Common examples of this category include:

(1) Psychoses with unusual features, e.g., monosymptomatic delusion of bodily change without accompanying impairment in functioning; persistent auditory hallucinations as the only disturbance; transient psychotic episodes associated with the menstrual cycle.
(2) 'Postpartum psychoses' that do not meet the criteria for an Organic Mental Disorder, Schizophreniform Disorder, Paranoid Disorder, or Affective Disorder.
(3) Psychoses that would be classified elsewhere except that the duration is less than two weeks, e.g., the symptomatology of a Schizophreniform Disorder, but lasting only three days and there is no precipitating psychosocial stressor.
(4) Psychoses about which there is inadequate information to make a more specific diagnosis. (This is preferable to Diagnosis Deferred, and can be changed if more information becomes available.)
(5) Psychoses with confusing clinical features that make a more specific diagnosis impossible.

COMMENTARY

Apart from the introduction of several axes for the systematic registration of various areas of disturbance and information, DSM–III (1980) contrasts with ICD–9 in its use of operationalized inclusion and exclusion criteria. Among the latter, point G excludes clear organicity and point F excludes 'the full depressive or manic syndrome (criteria A and B of major depressive or manic episode).' Were F to conclude with 'is not present,' evidence to the contrary would unequivocally exclude a paranoid disorder. Instead, F reads; 'Is either not present, developed after any psychotic symptoms, or was brief in duration relative to the duration of the psychotic symptoms'. Therefore, exclusion depends upon when a full affective syndrome appears and how long it lasts. Prolongation of the syndrome would not influence the diagnosis of a chronic paranoid disorder; however, it would certainly affect that of the shorter ones in an arbitrary fashion.
A further element of uncertainty crops up in the demarcation of

paranoid disorder to schizophrenia, whereby the criteria A for the latter exclude the former (see the corresponding section in Chapter B9 on schizophrenia). In this connexion we must once again look at the criteria for schizophrenia: judging how bizarre are the delusional phenomena (A1) for diagnostic purposes is problematical, as are delusional perceptions, one of Kurt Schneider's first rank symptoms. In theory, guidelines such as Bleulerian and Schneiderian criteria, illustrated through clear examples of schizophrenic autism and ambivalence on the one hand and bizarre delusional perceptions on the other, should enable one to arrive at a decision with relative ease. In daily clinical practice, however, such guidelines become obscured through interpretations that, in the authors' opinion, are too broad. As stated, for example, Bleulerian criteria are vigorous and unequivocal; one is astonished, therefore, to discover that in practice the majority of paranoid disorders, even when offering quite plausible delusional themes, are diagnosed as schizophrenia. Again, one may very well suspect that individual terms of even the apparently rigorous and clearly conceived DSM–III criteria for schizophrenia receive varying interpretations depending upon region and school. The differential diagnostic considerations in DSM–III concerning paranoid disorders resemble in part those of ICD–9. Here also attention is called to the possible occurrence of loosening of associations, 'prominent hallucinations' and thematic variation in delusional phenomena (bizarre versus non-bizarre). Paranoid personality disorders (300.00, to be encoded on axis 2) are explicitly demarcated from paranoid disorders.

The diagnostic criteria for a paranoid disorder are restricted to non-bizarre delusional themes such as persecution or jealousy (A). Criterion B results implicitly from the exclusion criterion D. When hallucinations occur, deciding whether they are 'prominent' (criterion E) is also arbitrary; if all other criteria for a paranoid illness are present as well, a paranoid disorder such as paranoia or a shared paranoid or acute paranoid disorder may not be diagnosed, at the most only 297.9, atypical paranoid disorder, or eventually 298.90, atypical psychosis, as a residual category.

The exclusion criterion D for paranoid disorder is unequivocally formulated ('none of the symptoms of criterion A of schizophrenia'), just as for organic disorders. For affective disorders the situation is somewhat more complicated because allowance is made for their occurrence when following psychotic symptoms (to prevent therapy-induced or reactive depressions from being used as exclusion criteria) or when relatively brief (see above).

Paranoia (297.10) is defined by means of the seven criteria for paranoid disorder; also required are a minimal duration of six months for the delusional symptomatology and the exclusion of a shared paranoid disorder. A small inconsistency occurs because point A of the diagnostic criteria for paranoid disorder refers to persistent delusions of persecution or jealousy, whereas point B of the diagnostic criteria for paranoia simply refers to a persecutory system. This is surely an oversight, for in the introductory paragraph on paranoia one reads that chronic forms of 'conjugal paranoia' are to be rated here. On the other hand, an upper age limit for illness onset, as given in the criteria of Winokur (1977) and Kendler (1980a) for example, does not exist; therefore, one is able to classify with certainty at least a part of the paranoid states which appear during involution.

The criteria for shared paranoid disorder (297.30) correspond to the general diagnostic criteria for a paranoid disorder restricted to the theme of persecution. In contrast to paranoia there is no requirement that the delusion should last at least six months. Disregarding the restriction of themes and the minimal duration of one week, the criteria are identical with those of ICD–9.

For the acute paranoid disorder (298.30) the six-month criterion of paranoia is not required, and the introductory sentences indicate possible connexions between outbreak of the disorder and important life-events (immigrants, refugees, prisoners of war, inductees into military services, and so on) without making the latter obligatory. By and large, this category corresponds to the reactive paranoid psychoses of Scandinavian nomenclature (see Chapter E2).

For paranoid syndromes which cannot be classified among the schizo-phrenic or manic-depressive disorders and do not correspond to any of the criteria for paranoid disorders mentioned so far, there is a residual category called 'atypical paranoid disorder' (297.90). Cases such as the above-mentioned, which manifest 'prominent hallucinations' in addition to fulfilling all other criteria for paranoia, may be classified here, possibly also those characterized by chronic, stable delusional syndromes lacking in rich, productive symptomatology, but exhibiting themes other than persecution and jealousy.

In clinical practice, inevitably there are cases sometimes which still elude classification; for them, aside from the diagnostic possibility of schizoaffective disorder (see Chapter D6, 295.70), the residual category 298.90, atypical psychosis, was created. Patients manifesting more or less well-organized delusional syndromes would correspond to only the first example given.

A central feature distinguishing the criteria of DSM–III from those of ICD–9 is the former's restriction to two delusional themes. Kendler (1980b) questions the validity of this distinction. For the paranoid disorder concept DSM–III leans more heavily on the Bleulerian than on the Kraepelinian school, according to which it is also possible to accept even bizarre or fantastic delusional content with highly prominent halluci-nations as 'non-schizophrenic.'

Setting an illness onset-age limit of 45 years for schizophrenia creates a problem. One sees time and again somewhat older patients with no sign whatsoever of organic, presenile, or even senile psychoses who exhibit delusional syndromes that, on the whole, correspond to the DSM–III criteria for schizophrenia with the exception of the age stipulation. The paranoid disorders are too strictly conceived to include such cases, so that 298.90 remains as a catch-all, perhaps to an excessive degree, for these and other fully heterogeneous cases.

E7

Diagnostic and statistical manual of mental disorders, third edition, revised (DSM-III-R)

CRITERIA

Delusional (paranoid) disorder

297.10 Delusional (paranoid) disorder

A. Nonbizarre delusion(s) (i.e., involving situations that occur in real life, such as being followed, poisoned, infected, loved at a distance, having a disease, being deceived by one's spouse or lover) of at least one month's duration.

B. Auditory or visual hallucinations, if present are not prominent (as defined in Schizophrenia, A (1b)). [See Chapter B10.]

C. Apart from the delusion(s) or its ramifications, behavior is not obviously odd or bizarre.

D. If a Major Depressive or Manic syndrome has been present during the delusional disturbance, the total duration of all episodes of the mood syndrome has been brief relative to the total duration of the delusional disturbance.

E. Has never met criterion A for Schizophrenia, and it cannot be established that an organic factor initiated and maintained the disturbance. [See Chapter B10.]

> **Specify type:** The following types are based on the predominant delusional theme. If no single delusional theme predominates, specify as *Unspecified Type*.

Erotomanic type

Delusional Disorder in which the predominant theme of the delusion(s) is that a person, usually of higher status, is in love with the subject.

Source of criteria: Diagnostic and statistical manual of mental disorders, third edition, revised (DSM-III-R) (1987). Washington, DC: American Psychiatric Association.

Grandiose type

Delusional Disorder in which the predominant theme of the delusion(s) is one of inflated worth, power, knowledge, identity, or special relationship to a deity or famous person.

Jealous type

Delusional Disorder in which the predominant theme of the delusion(s) is that one's sexual partner is unfaithful.

Persecutory type

Delusional Disorder in which the predominant theme of the delusion(s) is that one (or someone to whom one is close) is being malevolently treated in some way. People with this type of Delusional Disorder may repeatedly take their complaints of being mistreated to legal authorities.

Somatic type

Delusional Disorder in which the predominant theme of the delusion(s) is that the person has some physical defect, disorder, or disease.

Unspecified type

Delusional Disorder that does not fit any of the previous categories, e.g., persecutory and grandiose themes without a predominance of either; delusions of reference without malevolent content.

Psychotic disorders not elsewhere classified

297.30 Induced psychotic disorder (shared paranoid disorder)

A. A delusion develops (in a second person) in the context of a close relationship with another person, or persons, with an already established delusion (the primary case).
B. The delusion in the second person is similar in content to that in the primary case.
C. Immediately before onset of the induced delusion, the second person did not have a psychotic disorder or the prodromal symptoms of Schizophrenia. [See Chapter B10.]

298.90 Psychotic disorder not otherwise specified (atypical psychosis)

Disorders in which there are psychotic symptoms (delusions, hallucinations, incoherence, marked loosening of associations, catatonic excitement or stupor, or grossly disorganized behavior) that do not meet the criteria for any other nonorganic psychotic disorder. This category should also be used for psychoses about which there is inadequate information to make a specific diagnosis. (This is preferable to 'Diagnosis Deferred,' and can be changed if more information becomes available.) This diagnosis is made only when it cannot be established that an organic factor initiated and maintained the disturbance.

Examples:

(1) psychoses with unusual features, e.g., persistent auditory hallucinations as the only disturbance
(2) postpartum psychoses that do not meet the criteria for an Organic Mental Disorder, psychotic Mood Disorder, or any other psychotic disorder
(3) psychoses with confusing clinical features that make a more specific diagnosis impossible

COMMENTARY

Simplifications and improvements have been introduced into the DSM-III-R (1987) sections for schizophrenic and paranoid disorders, both of which are relevant to this chapter.

The designation of the whole section has been changed. It was pointed out that 'the term "paranoid" has multiple other meanings' (DSM-III-R, p. 199), which is why the term 'delusional' shall replace it from now on.

The criteria A for schizophrenia are more clearly defined (see Chapter B10). Moreover the age stipulation (illness onset before age 45) no longer exists. On the one hand, this enables a better, sharper delimitation of delusional from schizophrenic disorders; on the other hand, late-onset illnesses, that fulfill the criteria A for schizophrenia and about which sufficient information is available, no longer have to be relegated to a residual category.

The DSM-III-R delusional disorder concept is no longer limited exclusively to delusions of persecution and jealousy, but has been broadened to include somatic, erotomanic, and grandiose delusions. Restrictions concerning hallucinations have also been eased. Whereas 'no prominent hallucinations' whatsoever were accepted under DSM-III (see Chapter E6), this stipulation is made in DSM-III-R only for auditory and optic phenomena; all other hallucinations may be admitted regardless of their intensity. No modifications have been introduced regarding the exclusion of schizophrenic and affective disorders.

An important rectification was made for the time span of the disorder: in contrast to the DSM-III diagnostic requirement that a paranoid disorder should last at least six months, a time span of only one month suffices.

Therefore, the new definition is appreciably broader than that of DSM-III (see Chapter E6), approaches the Kendlerian criteria (Kender, 1980*a*) (see Chapter E10), and should reduce the number of cases that are hard to classify despite adequate information. It also renders superfluous the formulation of an acute paranoid disorder (298.30), for which DSM-III requires a duration of one week to six months.

The DSM-III-R version for shared paranoid disorder (297.30), noted together with atypical psychosis (298.90) under 'psychotic disorders not elsewhere classified,' specifies the notion of induction more precisely, see criteria A–C.

The residual category, atypical psychosis (298.90) whose formulation differs little from that of DSM-III, will surely henceforth be reserved for a far smaller number of cases that are really hard to classify.

Taking everything into account the development of diagnostic formulations according to DSM-III-R represents a marked improvement and standardization compared with DSM-III (see Chapter E6). It would be an exaggeration to maintain that this indicates a rapprochement to the concept of non-schizophrenic paranoid psychoses formulated by Kraepelin in the 8th edition of his Textbook (1909–1915); yet, the new version is undoubtedly closer to clinical reality and in this respect finds support from recent research results (see Schanda, 1987).

E8

Present state examination (PSE)/CATEGO system

Class P+. paranoid psychoses

The chief symptoms are:

I delusions (other than first rank)
II hallucinations (other than auditory)

Class P?

I delusions of persecution or reference (in the absence of more diagnostic symptoms)
II 'partial' delusions

Source of criteria: Wing, J. K., Cooper, J. E. and Sartorius N. (1974) *Measurement and classification of psychiatric symptoms*. Cambridge: Cambridge University Press.

For information concerning the creation and development of the present state examination (PSE) and the computer program (CATEGO) processing the data of this semi-standardized interview, also regarding their application and relevant reliability investigations, the reader is referred to Chapter B13 in the section on schizophrenia.

For the chapter on non-schizophrenic paranoid psychoses there are two important points:

1. The precise description of the CATEGO class P (paranoid psychoses) on the basis of individual symptoms and syndromes

2. The differential diagnostic delimitation to other CATEGO classes (above all class S, schizophrenic psychoses)

The chief symptoms of class P+ are delusional symptoms (other than first rank symptoms) and hallucinations other than auditory. Therefore, P+ comprises patients with delusional phenomena and hallucinations that do not figure among the symptoms of classes S+, M+, or D+. There are close ties to the ICD-9 (1978) diagnoses 297.0, 298.2, 298.3, 298.9, and 299.

Class P? is the only uncertain psychotic class of relatively frequent occurrence. Characteristic symptoms are phenomena of persecution and prejudice without further symptoms of diagnostic relevance or partial delusions.

Class P showed a syndrome profile drawing the highest values in the syndrome groups 14 (delusions of persecution), 15 (delusions of reference), 6 (simple depression), 8 (general anxiety), 18 (visual hallucinations), 11 (affective flattening), 3 (incoherent speech), and 21 (slowness), not only in the international pilot study of schizophrenia (IPSS; WHO, 1973) but also in the US–UK study (Cooper *et al.*, 1972). Similarities to the syndrome profile of class S, which contains thought intrusion, thought broadcasting or withdrawal, delusions of control, voices discussing the patient in the third person or commenting on his/her thoughts or actions, other auditory hallucinations (not affectively based), and other delusions as characteristic symptoms, can be found markedly loading syndromes 24 (special features of depression), 6 (simple depression), 8 (general anxiety), 14 (delusions of persecution), 15 (delusions of reference), 21 (slowness), 3 (incoherent speech), and 11 (affective flattening).

Highly discriminating symptoms for the distinction between classes S+ and P+ are: voices speaking to the patient, voices discussing the patient, commenting voices, thought broadcasting, and delusions of control. All of them are cited among the first rank symptoms.

The 12 major CATEGO classes can be subdivided into 50 subclasses (see Wing *et al.*, 1974). These elements may be put together in various ways; for example, one may form a schizoaffective class and possibly subdivide it into manic and depressive subtypes.

It must be pointed out once again that the various CATEGO classes do not represent nosological diagnoses. As for the importance of the PSE/CATEGO system for research, see Chapter 13 in the section on schizophrenia.

E9

Winokur's diagnostic criteria for delusional disorder (paranoia)

1. All patients have to exhibit an unequivocal delusion
2. Such a delusion or delusions could have been present for any length of time
3. The delusions have to be related to events that were possible, however implausible
4. Does not meet any of the following exclusion criteria:

   a. The presence or suggestion of the presence of any hallucinations at any time

   b. Bizarre or fantastic delusions at any time

   c. Evidence of organic brain syndrome

   d. Illness beginning after the age of 60

   e. Meeting clear criteria for depression or mania

   f. Inappropriateness or marked flattening of affect

Source of criteria: Winokur, G. (1977) Delusional disorder (paranoia). *Compr. Psychiat.*, **18**, 511–21.

The investigations of Winokur and his associates were inspired by the observation that first-degree relatives of paranoid schizophrenics are less likely to suffer from schizophrenia than are those of non-paranoid schizophrenics, a circumstance already mentioned by Schulz (1932) and Kallmann (1938). Results led first to the establishment of criteria that were to distinguish between paranoid and non-paranoid forms of schizophrenia (Tsuang and Winokur, 1974), then ultimately to the criteria for paranoia cited at the beginning of the chapter. The criteria are supposed to register any kind of delusional syndrome clearly lacking signs of schizophrenic, affective, or organic disorders. Winokur (1977) initially found that schizophrenia occurred more often in first-degree relatives of patients with delusional disorders than in those of manic-depressives and about as often as in those of schizophrenics; however, this diagnosis of schizophrenia included chronic cases of paranoid psychoses as well. After exclusion of these cases from the schizophrenia group, schizophrenia was found to occur about as often in first-degree relatives of paranoid patients as in those of patients with affective disorders. Kendler and Hays (1981) were able to duplicate this observation.

Winokur requires no minimal duration of symptoms, in contrast to DSM-III for example, (see Chapter E6), but establishes an age limit of 60 years for illness onset, as does Kendler (1980a). The exclusion criterion for organic or affective disorders (4c, 4e) is not as strictly formulated as in DSM-III. Paranoid disorder is, on the one hand, less strictly demarcated to schizophrenia than in DSM-III because Winokur, although excluding bizarre delusional content, does not limit the possible delusional themes to those of persecution and jealousy alone. On the other hand, Winokur is much stricter concerning the occurrence of hallucinatory phenomena when he explicitly introduces 'the presence or suggestion of the presence of any hallucinations at any time' as an exclusion criterion. For the most part, patients who are diagnosed as having delusional disorder under Winokur's criteria could also be diagnosed as having simple paranoid psychosis (297.0) or paranoia (297.1) according to ICD-9, paranoid disorder (297) according to DSM-III, or simple delusional disorder under Kendler's (1980a) criteria.

E10

Kendler's diagnostic criteria for delusional disorder (paranoid psychosis)

Simple delusional disorder

1. Onset of illness before age 60
2. Nonbizarre delusions of any type and/or persistent, pervasive ideas of reference lasting at least 2 weeks
3. A full affective syndrome, either depressed or manic, was absent when the patient was delusional
4. There were no symptoms suggestive of schizophrenia, including prominent thought disorder, inappropriate affect, patently bizarre delusions, or Schneiderian symptoms
5. Symptoms suggestive of an acute or chronic brain syndrome are absent
6. Absence of persistent hallucinations of any kind

Hallucinatory delusional disorder

1. Meets criteria 1–5 for simple delusional disorder
2. Presence of hallucinations of any kind except those described by Schneider as indicative of schizophrenia (i.e., voices commenting, discussing patient, or repeating patient's thoughts)

Source of criteria: Kendler, K. S. (1980*a*) The nosologic validity of paranoia (simple delusional disorder): a review. *Arch. Gen. Psychiat*, **37**, 699–706.

COMMENTARY

Kendler's (1980*a*) diagnostic criteria for delusional disorder are to be regarded as a further development of Winokur's criteria (1977). Like the latter they are based on the assumption that this illness entity occupies a special position lying outside the realm of schizophrenia on the one hand and on the observation that its genetic determination is variable on the other.

Affiliation to the other criteria employed in the United States (DSM–III–R and, precisely, Winokur; see Chapters E7 and E9) is evident. Kendler requires, as does Winokur, an illness onset before age 60 and a minimal duration of two weeks (DSM–III requires one week). Exclusion criteria for organic illnesses are identical with those of Winokur; however, for affective disorders Kendler follows a different path: leaning heavily on point F of the DSM–III criteria for paranoid disorders, he stipulates only that an affective syndrome may not occur 'when the patient was delusional;' that is, its presence at any other time does not rule out the diagnosis. In contrast to DSM–III any delusional theme is acceptable, as long as it is not bizarre. Kendler (1980*b*) himself argued against the DSM–III restriction to the delusional themes of persecution and jealousy; he showed, by means of three investigations, that a delusional theme has no influence whatsoever on the course and outcome of an illness – an argument that, of course, may also be used against his own restriction (bizarreness). As symptoms suggestive of schizophrenia, in addition to the bizarre delusional content already mentioned, he suggested thought disorders and inappropriate affect, hereby agreeing with DSM–III entirely and with the Scandinavian school in part (see, Chapter E2). He included also Schneiderian symptoms among the exclusion criteria. However, this is questionable, since their lack of predictive capacity for the diagnosis of schizophrenia has already been demonstrated several times on the basis of illness course investigations (Carpenter *et al.*, 1973*b*; Strauss and Carpenter, 1977; WHO, 1979; Stephens *et al.*, 1980, 1982; Schanda *et al.*, 1984). Questionable above all in this respect is the symptom of delusional perception, whose use in diagnostic decision-making may lead to non-uniformity, owing to its unclear formulation and ubiquitous occurrence. Contrary to Winokur (1977), Kendler recognized the importance of identifying non-schizophrenic delusional psychoses characterized also by the presence of hallucinations, albeit not in the form of first rank symptoms. (In this respect a compromise is made in DSM–III by allowing hallucinations but stipulating that they may not be 'dominating'). For this reason he introduced along with his classification of simple delusional disorder, the category of hallucinatory delusional disorder.

An investigation of family histories (Kendler and Hays, 1981) showed that the criteria for simple delusional disorder are clearly capable of identifying a group of paranoid psychotics as an entity distinct from schizophrenia.

F

BIBLIOGRAPHY

Note: Designations at end of each bibliographic entry indicate where the reference is relevant.

Abou-Saleh, M. T. and Coppen, A. (1983) A classification of depression and response to antidepressive therapies. *Brit. J. Psychiat.*, **143**, 601–3. [C12]

Abou-Saleh, M. T. and Coppen, A. (1984) Classification of depressive illnesses. Clinicopsychological correlates. *J. Aff. Disord.*, **6**, 53–66. [C12]

Abrams, R. and Taylor, M. A. (1978) A rating scale for emotional blunting. *Am. J. Psychiat.*, **135**, 226–9. [B15]

Abrams, R., Taylor, M. A. and Gaztanaga, P. (1974) Manic-depressive illness and paranoid schizophrenia. A phenomenological, family history and treatment-response study. *Arch. Gen. Psychiat.*, **31**, 640–2. [C11]

Andreasen, N. C. (1979) Affective flattening and criteria for schizophrenia. *Am. J. Psychiat.*, **136**, 944–7. [B14, B15]

Andreasen, N. C., Scheftner, W., Reich, T., Hirschfeld, R. M. A., Endicott, J. and Keller, M. B. (1986) The validation of the concept of endogenous depression. *Arch. Gen. Psychiat.*, **43**, 246–51. [C12]

Angst, J. (1966) *Zur Ätiologie und Nosologie endogener depressiver Psychosen.* Heidelberg, New York, Berlin: Springer. [A, C5, C10]

Angst, J. (1986) The course of schizoaffective disorders. In Marneros, A. and Tsuang, M. T. (eds.) *Schizoaffective psychoses.* Berlin, Heidelberg, New York: Springer. [D3, D4]

Ansseau, M., Cerfontaine, J.-L., von Frenckell, R., Charles, G., Papart, P. and Franck, G. (1987) L'index de Newcastle pour le diagnostic de dépression endogène. *L'Encéphale*, **13**, 67–72. [C12]

Arnold, O. H., Gastager, H. and Hofmann, G. (1965) Klinische, Psychopathologische und Biochemische Untersuchungen an Legierungspsychosen. *Wr. Zeitschr. Nervenheilk.*, **4**, 301–61. [D]

Astrachan, B. M., Harrow, M., Adler, D., Brauer, L., Schwartz, A. and Schwartz, C. (1972) A checklist for the diagnosis of schizophrenia. *Brit. J. Psychiat.*, **121**, 529–39. [B11]

Astrup, C., Fossum, A. and Holmboe, R. (1962) *Prognosis in functional psychoses. Clinical, social and genetic aspects.* Springfield, Ill: Thomas. [E2]

Astrup, C. and Noreik, K. (1966) *Functional psychoses: diagnostic and prognostic models.* Springfield, Ill: Thomas. [E2]

Baillarger J. (1854) De la folie á double forme. *Ann. Med. Psychol.*, **6**, 369–84. [A, C10]

Ballet, G. (1911) La psychose hallucinatoire chronique. *L'Encéphale*, **6**, 401–11. [B16]

Bebbington, P., Hurry, J., Tennant, C., Sturt, E. and Wing, J. K. (1981) Epidemiology of mental disorders in Camberwell. *Psychol. Med.*, **11**, 561–79. [B13, C9]

Bech, P., Allerup, P., Gram, L. F., Krag-Sørensen, P., Rafaelsen, O. J., Reisby, N., Vestergaard, P. and the Danish University Antidepressant Group (DUAG). (1988) The diagnostic melancholia scale (DMS): dimensions of endogenous and reactive depression with relationship to the Newcastle scales. *J. of Affective Disorders*, **14**, 161–70. [C12]

Bech, P., Gjerris, A., Andersen, J. Bøjholm, S., Kramp, P., Bolwig, T. G., Kastrup, M., Clemmesen, L. and Rafaelsen, O. J. (1983) The melancholia scale and the Newcastle scales. Item combinations and interobserver reliability. *Brit. J. Psychiat.*, **143**, 58–63. [C12]

Bech, P., Gram, L. F., Reisby, N. and Rafaelsen, O. J. (1980) The WHO Depression Scale. Relationship to the Newcastle scales. *Acta Psychiat. Scand.*, **62**, 140–53. [C12]

Berner, P. (1965) Das paranoide Syndrom. *Monographie aus dem Gesamtgebiete der Neurologie und Psychiatrie*, **110**, Berlin: Springer. [B14, C10]

Berner, P. (1969) Der Lebensabend der Paranoiker. *Wien Z. Nerv. Heilk.*, **27**, 115–61. [B14, C10]

Berner, P. (1982) Unter welchen Bedingungen lassen weitere Verlaufs-forschungen noch neue Erkenntnisse über die endogenen Psychosen erwarten? *Psychiat. Clin.*, **15**, 3:97–123. [A, B14, C10]

Berner, P. (1983) Die Unterteilung der endogenen Psychosen: Differential-diagnostik oder Differentialtypologie. In Gross, G. and Schüttler, R. (eds.) *Empirische Forschung in der Psychiatrie.* Stuttgart, New York: Schattauer. [B15]

Berner, P., Gabriel, E., Katschnig, H., Kieffer, W., Koehler, K., Lenz, G. and Simhandl, Ch. (1983a) *Diagnostic criteria for schizophrenic and affective psychoses.* Published by the World Psychiatric Assocation on the occasion of the VII World Congress of Psychiatry, Vienna, 1983. Washington, DC: Printed and distributed by the American Psychiatric Press. [Preface, C12, D, E1]

Berner, P., Gabriel, E., Kieffer, W. and Schanda, H. (1986a) Paranoid psychoses: new aspects of classification coming from the Vienna Research Group. *Psychopathology*, **19**, 16–29. [E, E1]

Berner, P. and Katschnig, H. (1983) Principles of 'multiaxial' classification in psychiatry as a basis of modern methodology. In Helgason, T. (ed.) *Methods in evaluation of psychiatric treatment.* Cambridge: Cambridge Univ. Press. [A]

Berner, P., Katschnig, H. and Lenz, G. (1983b) DSM–III in German-speaking countries. In Spitzer, R. L., Williams, J. B. W. and Skodol, A. E. (eds.) *International perspectives on DSM–III.* Washington, DC: American Psychiatric Press. [A]

Berner, P., Katschnig, H. and Lenz, G. (1983c) Sémiologie et nosologie. *Acta Psychiat. Belgica.*, **83**, 181–96. [A, B14, C10]

Berner, P., Katschnig, H. and Lenz, G. (1986b) First rank symptoms and Bleuler's basic symptoms: new results in applying the polydiagnostic approach. *Psychopathology*, **19**, 244–52. [A]

Berner, P., Katschnig, H. and Lenz, G. (1986c) The polydiagnostic approach in research on schizophrenia. In Freedman, A., Brotman, R., Silverman, I. and Hutson, D. (eds.) *Science, practice and social policy: issues in classifying mental disorders*. New York: Human Sciences Press, 70–91. [A]

Berner, P. and Lenz, G. (1986) Definitions of schizoaffective psychosis: Mutual concordance and relationship to schizophrenia and affective disorder. In Marneros, A. and Tsuang, M. T. (eds.) *Schizoaffective Psychoses*. Springer: Berlin. [D3]

Birnbaum, K. (1908) *Psychosen mit Wahnbildung und wahnhafte Einbildungen bei Degenerierten*. Halle: Marhold. [E2]

Bland, R. C. and Orn, H. (1980) Prediction of long-term outcome from presenting symptoms in schizophrenia. *J. Clin. Psychiat.*, **41**, 85–8. [B11]

Bleuler, E. (1911) *Dementia praecox oder Gruppe der Schizophrenien*. Leipzig, Wien: Deuticke. Reprint München: Minerva Publikation (1978). English edition *Dementia praecox or the group of schizophrenias*. Translated by Zinkin, J. New York: Intern. Univ. Press (1950). [A, B1, B2, B4, B5, B9, B17, E]

Bleuler, E. (1983) *Lehrbuch der Psychiatrie*. 15.Aufl. neubearbeitet von M. Bleuler. Berlin: Springer. [B2, B3]

Bleuler, M. (1972) *Die schizophrenen Geistesstörungen im Lichte langjähriger Kranken- und Familiengeschichten*. Stuttgart, Thieme. [B2, B3]

Bleuler, M. (1981) Einzelkrankheiten in der Schizophrenie-Gruppe. In Huber, G. (ed.) *Schizophrenie, Stand und Entwicklungstendenzen der Forschung*. Stuttgart: Schattauer. [B2]

Bleuler, M., Huber, G., Gross, G. and Schüttler, R. (1976) Der langfristige Verlauf schizophrener Psychosen. Gemeinsame Ergebnisse zweier Untersuchungen. *Nervenarzt*, **47**, 477–81. [B2, B3]

Bochnik, H. J., and Gärtner-Huth, C. (1982) Schizoaffektive-gleich atypische-phasische Psychosen. In Huber, G. (ed.) *Das ärztliche Gespräch Heft*, **36**. Köln: Troponwerke. [D]

Boeters, U. (1971) *Die oneiroiden Emotionspsychosen. Klinische Studie als Beitrag zur Differentialdiagnose atypischer Psychosen*. Basel, München, Paris, London, New York, Sydney: Karger. [D]

Bonhoeffer, K. (1907) *Klinische Beiträge zur Lehre von den Degenerationspsychosen*. Halle: Marhold. [E2]

Brockington, I. F., Kendell, R. E. and Leff, J. P. (1978) Definitions of schizophrenia and prediction of outcome. *Psychol. Med.*, **8**, 387–98. [A, B4, B7, B11, B12]

Brockington, I. F. and Leff, J. P. (1979) Schizo-affective psychosis: definitions and incidence. *Psychol. Med.*, **9**, 91–9. [D, D1]

Brockington, I. F. and Meltzer, H. Y. (1983) The nosology of schizoaffective psychosis. *Psychiatric Developments*, **4**, 317–38. [D5, D7]

Brockington, I. F., Perris, C. and Kendell, R. E. (1982a) The course and outcome of cycloid psychosis. *Psychol. Med.*, **12**, 97–105. [D2]

Brockington, I. F., Perris, C. and Meltzer, H. Y. (1982b) Cycloid psychoses. Diagnosis and heuristic value. *J. Nerv. Ment. Dis.*, **17**, 11, 651–6. [D2]

Carlson, G. A. and Goodwin, F. K. (1973) The stages of mania. A longitudinal analysis of the manic episode. *Arch. Gen. Psychiat.*, **28**, 221–8. [A]

Carney, M. W. P., Reynolds, E. H. and Sheffield, B. F. (1986) Prediction of outcome in depressive illness by the Newcastle diagnosis scale. *Brit. J. Psychiat.*, **150**, 43–8. [C12]

Carney, M. W. P., Roth, M. and Garside, R. F. (1965) The diagnosis of depressive syndromes and the prediction of E.C.T. response. *Brit. J. Psychiat.*, **III**, 659–74. [A, C12, C13]

Carney, M. W. P. and Sheffield, B. F. (1972) Depression and the Newcastle scales. Their relationship to Hamilton's scale. *Brit. J. Psychiat.*, **121**, 35–40. [C12]

Carpenter, W. T. (1976) Current diagnostic concepts in schizophrenia. *Am. J. Psychiat.*, **133**, 172–7. [B12]

Carpenter, W. T. jr, and Strauss, J. S. (1974) Cross cultural evaluation of Schneider's first rank symptoms of schizophrenia: a report from the international pilot study of schizophrenia. *Am. J. Psychiat.*, **133**, 682–7. [B3]

Carpenter, W. T., Strauss, J. S. and Bartko, J. J. (1973a) Flexible system for the diagnosis of schizophrenia: Report from the WHO International Pilot Study of Schizophrenia. *Science*, **182**, 1275–8. [B12]

Carpenter, W. T. jr, Strauss, J. S. and Muleh, S. (1973b) Are there pathognomonic symptoms in schizophrenia? An empiric investigation of Schneider's first rank symptoms. *Arch. Gen. Psychiat.* **28**, 847–52. [B3, E10]

Checkly, S. A. (1979) Corticosteroid and growth hormone responses to methylamphetamine in depressive illness. *Psychol. Med.*, **9**, 107–15. [C12]

Clayton, P. J. (1982) Schizoaffective disorder. *J. Nerv. Ment. Dis.*, **11**, 646–50. [D5, D7]

Clérambault, G. de. (1942) *Oeuvre psychiatrique*, première edition. Paris: PUF. [B16]

Cooper, B., Kendell, R. E., Gurland, B. J., Sharpe, L., Copeland, J. R. M. and Simon, R. (1972) *Psychiatric diagnosis in New York and London*. London: Oxford University Press. [B13, C9, E8]

Coppen, A., Alou-Saleh, M., Milln, P., Metcalfe, M., Harwood, J. and Bailey, J. (1983) Dexamethasone suppression test in depression and other psychiatric illness. *Brit. J. Psychiat.*, **142**, 498–501. [C12]

Coryell, W. and Tsuang, M. T. (1982) DSM–III schizophreniform disorder. Comparisons with schizophrenia and affective disorder. *Arch. Gen. Psychiat.* **39**, 66–9. [B9, C7]

Cutting, J. C., Clare, A. W. and Mann, A. H. (1978) Cycloid psychosis: An investigation of the diagnostic concept. *Psychol. Med.*, **8**, 637–48. [D2]

Dam, H., Mellerup, E. T. and Rafaelsen, O. J. (1985) The dexamethasone suppression test in depression. *J. of Affective Disorders*, **8**, 95–103. [C12]

Davidson, J., Lipper, S., Zung, W. W. K., Strickland, R., Krischnan, R. and Mahorney, S. (1984a) Validation of four definitions of melancholia by the dexamethasone suppression test. *Am. J. Psychiat.*, **141**, 1220–3. [A, C12]

Davidson, J. R. T., McLeod, M. N., Turnbull, C. D., White, H. L. and Feuer, E. J. (1980) Platelet monoamine oxidase activity and the classification of depression. *Arch. Gen. Psychiat.*, **37**, 771–3. [C12]

Davidson, J. R. T., Strickland, R., Turnbull, C. D., Belyea, M. and Miller,

R. D. (1984*b*) The Newcastle endogenous depression diagnostic index (NEDDI): validity and reliability. *Acta Psychiat. Scand.*, **69**, 220–30. [C 12]

Diagnostic and statistical manual of mental disorders, second edition (DSM–II) (1968) Washington, DC: American Psychiatric Assocation. [B11, B15]

Diagnostic and statistical manual of mental disorders, third edition (DSM–III) (1980) Washington, DC: American Psychiatric Association. [B9, B16, C7, D6, E, E1, E4, E5, E6, E7, E9]

Diagnostic and statistical manual of mental disorders, third edition, revised (DSM–III–R) (1987) Washington, DC: American Psychiatric Association. [A, B10, C8, D, D7, E, E1, E5, E7]

Endicott, J., Nee, J., Fleiss, J., Cohen, J., Williams, J. B. W. and Simon, R. (1982) Diagnostic criteria for schizophrenia. Reliabilities and agreements between systems. *Arch. Gen. Psychiat.*, **39**, 884–9. [A, B7, B9, B11, B12]

Endicott, J. and Spitzer, R. L. (1978) A diagnostic interview: The schedule for affective disorders and schizophrenia. *Arch. Gen. Psychiat.*, **35**, 837–44. [B8, C6]

Faergemann, P. (1963) *Psychogenic psychoses. A description and follow-up of psychoses following psychological stress.* London: Butterworths, 1963 [D]

Falret, J. P. (1854) De la folie circulaire. *Bulletin de l'Academie de Médecine*, **19**, 382–398. [A]

Feighner, J. P. (1979) The nosology and phenomenology of primary affective disorders. In Obiols *et al.* (eds.) *Biological psychiatry today, proceedings of the 2nd world congress on biological psychiatry, Barcelona, 1978.* Amsterdam, New York, Oxford: Elsevier/North Holland Biomedical Press. [B11, C5]

Feighner, J. P. (1981) Nosology of primary affective disorders and application to clinical research. *Acta Psychiat. Scand.* (Suppl. 190), **63**, 29–41. [C5]

Feighner, J. P., Robins, E., Guze, S. B., Woodruff, R. A., Winokur, G. and Munoz, R. (1972) Diagnostic criteria for use in psychiatric research. *Arch. Gen. Psychiat.*, **26**, 57–63. [B7, B8, B9, C, C5, C6, D5]

Feinberg, M. and Carroll, B. J. (1982) Separation of subtypes of depression using discriminant analysis. I. Separation of unipolar endogenous depression from non-endogenous depression. *Brit. J. Psychiat.*, **140**, 384–391. [C12]

Feinberg, M. and Carroll, B. J. (1983) Separation of bipolar endogenous depression from non-endogenous ('neurotic') depression *J. Aff. Disord.*, **5**, 129–139. [C12]

Fenton, W. S., Mosher, L. R. and Matthews, S. N. (1981) Diagnosis of schizophrenia: A critical view of current diagnostic systems. *Schiz. Bull.*, **7**, 453–76. [B7, B8, B9, B11, B12]

Fish, F. (1967) *Clinical psycopathology.* Bristol: J. Wright [B15]

Fox, H. A. (1981) The DSM–III concept of schizophrenia. *Brit. J. Psychiat.*, **138**, 60–3. [B9, C7]

Gabriel, E. (1977) *Der langfristige verlauf von Spätschizophrenien. Zugleich ein Beitrag zum langen Verlauf von Wahnbildungen der Lebensmitte.* Bibliotheca Psychiatrica 156. Basel: Karger, [B14, C10]

Gaupp, R. (1910) Über paranoische Veranlagung und abortive Paranoia. *Allg. Z. Psychiat.*, **67**, 317–21. [A, E]

Giljarowskij, W. A. (1954) Lehrbuch der Psychiatrie. Moskau. Quoted by

Lustig, B. (1957) *Neue Forschungen in der Psychiatrie*. Berichte des Osteuropa-Institutes an der freien Universität Berlin, Heft 31. [B17]

Glossary (1974) *Glossary of mental disorders and guide to their classification for use in conjunction with the international classification of diseases*, eighth revision. Geneva: WHO. [B5, C2]

Gurney, C. (1971) *Diagnostic scales for affective disorders*. Abstract* (p. 330) from the Proceedings of the V World Congress of Psychiatry. Mexico City. [A, C12]

Gurney, C., Roth, M., Garside, R. F., Kerr, T. A. and Shapira, K. (1972) Studies in the classification of affective disorders. The relationship between anxiety states and depressive illness – II. *Brit. J. Psychiat.*, **121**, 162–6. [C12]

Haier, R. J. (1980). The diagnosis of schizophrenia: A review of recent developments. *Schiz. Bull.*, **6**, 417–28. [B7]

Hecker, E. (1871) Die Hebephrenie. *Virchows Arch. Path. Anat.*, **52**, 394–429. [B1]

Helmchen, H. (1975) Schizophrenia: Diagnostic concepts in the ICD 8. In Lader, M. H. (ed.) Studies of schizophrenia. *Brit. J. Psychiat.*, Special Publication **10**. [B5]

Helzer, J. E., Brockington, I. F. and Kendell, R. E. (1981) Predictive validity of DSM–III and Feighner definitions of schizophrenia. A comparison with Research Diagnostic Criteria and CATEGO. *Arch. Gen. Psychiat.*, **38**, 791–8. [A, B9, C7]

Helzer, J. E., Clayton, P. J., Pambakian, R. *et al.*, (1978) Concurrent diagnostic validity of a structured psychiatric interview. *Arch. Gen. Psychiat.*, **35**, 849–53. [B7]

Hoche, A. (1912) Die Bedeutung der Symptomenkomplexe in der Psychiatrie. *Zbl. ges Neurol. Psychiat.*, **12**, 540–51. [B14, C10, E]

Holden, N. L. (1983) Depression and the Newcastle scale. Their relationship to the dexamethasone suppression test. *Brit. J. Psychiat.*, **142**, 505–7. [C12]

Holland J. and Shakhmatova-Pavlova, I. V. (1977) Concept and classification of schizophrenia in the Soviet Union. *Schizophrenia Bulletin*, **3**, No. 2, 277–87. [B17]

ICD 8th Revision (1967) *WHO manual of the international statistical classification of diseases*, V (1965 revision), Geneva: WHO. [B5, C2, D3, E3]

ICD 9th Revision (1978) *Mental disorders: glossary and guide to their classification in accordance with the ninth revision of the international classification of diseases*. Geneva: WHO. [A, B5, C3, D3, E, E1, E3, E4, E5, E6, E8]

ICD–10 (1989a) *1989 draft of Chapter V, categories F00–F99/mental and behavioral disorders. Clinical descriptions and diagnostic guidelines*. April 1989. Division of Mental Health. Geneva: WHO. [A, B6, C4, D4, E1, E5]

ICD–10 (1989b) *1989 draft of chapter V, categories F00–F99/mental and behavioral disorders. Diagnostic criteria for research* (April 1989 draft for field trials). Division of Mental Health. Geneva: WHO. [A, B6, C4, D4, E5]

Institut National de la Santé et de la Recherche Médicale, section Psychiatrie (INSERM) (1968) Classification française des troubles mentaux. *Bull. Institut nat Santé Recherche*, méd **24**, suppl. no 2. [B16, C13]

---

* The original paper could not be found in the Proceedings of the Congress.

Janzarik. W. (1959) *Dynamische Grundkonstellationen in endogenen Psychosen.* Second edition. Berlin, Göttingen, Heidelberg: Springer. [A, B14 , B17, C10]

Jaspers, K. (1913) *Allgemeine Psychopathologie.* 1. Aufl Berlin. Heidelberg: Springer. [A, D3, E2]

Jaspers, K. (1946) *Allgemeine Psychopathologie.* 8. Aufl Berlin, Heidelberg, New York: Springer. [A]

Jaspers, K. (1963) *General Psychopathology.* Chicago: University of Chicago Press. [A, B14, B15, C6, C9, C10, C11, D3]

Jaspers, K. (1973) *Allgemeine Psychopathologie.* 9. Aufl Berlin, Heidelberg, New York: Springer. (E2)

Johanson E. (1964) Mild paranoia. Description and analysis of 52 inpatients from an open department for mental cases. *Acta Psychiat. Scand.*, Suppl. **177**. [E2]

Jung, R. (1952) Zur Klinik und Pathogenese der Depressionen. *Zbl. ges Neurol. psychiat.*, **119**, 163. [A]

Kahlbaum, K. L. (1874) *Die Katatonie oder das Spannungsirresein.* Berlin: Hirschwald. [B1]

Kallmann, F. (1938) *The genetics of schizophrenia.* New York: J. J. Augustin. [E9]

Kasanin J. (1933) The acute schizoaffective psychoses. *Am. J. Psychiat.*, **13**, 97–126 [A, B17, D, D1]

Katona, C. L. E., Aldridge, C. R., Roth, M. and Hyde, J. (1987) The dexamethasone suppression test and prediction of outcome in patients reciving ECT. *Brit. J. Psychiat.*, **150**, 315–18. [C12]

Katschnig, H. (1984*a*) Der polydiagnostische Ansatz in der psychiatrischen Forschung. In Hopf, A. and Beckmann, H. (Hrsg.) *Forschungen zur biologischen Psychiatrie.* Berlin, Heidelberg, New York: Springer. [A]

Katschnig, H. (1984*b*) Inferring Causes: some constraints in the social psychiatry of depression. Commentary to the article by Bebbington, P. E. *Integrative Psychiatry*, **2**, 77–9. [A, C9]

Katschnig, H. and Berner, P. (1985) The polydiagnostic approach in psychiatric research. In ADAMHA/WHO: *Mental disorders, alcohol and drug-related problems: international perspectives on their diagnosis and classification.* Amsterdam: Elsevier. [A]

Katschnig, H., Brandl-Nebehay, A., Fuchs-Robetin, G., Seelig, P., Eichberger, G., Strobl, R. and Sint, P. P. (1981) *Lebensverändernde Ereignisse, psychosoziale Dispositionen und depressive Verstimmungszustände.* Vienna: Psych. Univ. Clinic. [A]

Katschnig, H., Lenz, G., Musalek, M. Nutzinger, D., Schanda, H. and Simhandl, Ch. (1987) *The 'polydiagnostic system – 2 (PS2).'* Vienna: Psych. Univ. Clinic. [A]

Katschnig, H., Nutzinger, D. and Schanda, H. (1986*a*) Validating depressive subtypes. In Hippius, H., Klerman, G. and Matussek, N. (eds.): *New results in depression research.* Berlin, Heidelberg, New York: Springer. [A]

Katschnig, H., Pakesch, G. and Egger-Zeidner, E. (1986*b*) Life stress and depressive subtypes: a review of present diagnostic criteria and recent research results. In Katschnig, H. (ed.) *Life events and psychiatric disorders–controversial issues.* Cambridge: Cambridge Univ. Press. [A]

Katschnig, H. and Seelig, P. (1985) The polydiagnostic approach in psychiatric research on depression. In Pichot, P., Berner, P., Wolf R. and Thau, K. (eds.) *Psychiatry – The state of the art*, Vol 1, Proceedings of the 7th World Congress of Psychiatry, Vienna, 1983. New York: Plenum Publishing Corp. [A]

Katschnig, H. and Simhandl, Ch. (1986) New developments in the classification and diagnosis of functional mental disorders. *Psychopathology*, **19**, 219–35. [A]

Kendell, R. E. (1975) *The role of diagnosis in psychiatry*. Oxford: Blackwell Scientific Publications. [C12]

Kendell, R. E. (1976) The classification of depressions: a review of contemporary confusion. *Brit. J. Psychiat.*, **129**, 15–28. [C12]

Kendell, R. E. (1982) The choice of diagnostic criteria for biological research. *Arch Gen Psychiat*, **39**, 1334–9. [A]

Kendell, R. E. (1986) The relationship of schizoaffective illnesses to schizophrenic and affective disorders. In Marneros, A. and Tsuang, M. T. (eds.) *Schizoaffective psychoses*. Berlin, Heidelberg, New York: Springer. [D2, D5]

Kendell, R. E., Brockington, I. F. and Leff, J. (1979) Prognostic implications of six alternative definitions of schizophrenia. *Arch Gen. Psychiat.*, **36**, 25–31. [B4, B8, B11, B12]

Kendler, K. S. (1980*a*) The nosologic validity of paranoia (simple delusional disorder): a review. *Arch. Gen. Psychiat.*, **37**, 699–706. [E, E1, E5, E6, E7, E9, E10]

Kendler, K. S. (1980*b*) Are there delusions specific for paranoid disorders vs. schizophrenia? *Schiz. Bull.*, **6**, 1–3. [E6, E10]

Kendler, K. S. and Hays, P. (1981) Paranoid psychosis (delusional disorder) and schizophrenia. *Arch. Gen. Psychiat.*, **38**, 547–51. [E9, E10]

Kerr, T. A., Roth, M., Schapira, K. and Gurney, C. (1972) The assessment and prediction of outcome in affective disorders. *Brit. J. Psychiat.*, **121**, 167–74. [C12]

Kiloh, L. G., and Garside, R. F. (1963) The independence of neurotic depression and endogenous depression. *Brit. J. Psychiat.*, **109**, 451–63. [C12]

Klein, D. F. (1974) Endogenomorphic depression: a conceptual and terminological revision. *Arch. Gen. Psychiat.*, **31**, 447–54. [B14]

Kleist, K. (1928) Über zykloide, paranoide und epileptoide Psychosen und über die Frage der Degenerationspsychosen. *Schweiz. Arch. Gen. Neurochir. Psychiat.*, **23**, 3–37. [D, D2, E1]

Klerman, G. L. (1972) Clinical research in depression. In Zubin, J. and Freyhan, F. (eds.) *Disorders of mood*. Baltimore, London: John Hopkins Press. [C10]

Koehler, K. (1979) First rank symptoms of schizophrenia: questions concerning clinical boundaries. *Brit. J. Psychiat.*, **34**, 236–48. [A]

Kolle, K. (1931) *Die primäre Verrücktheit. Psychopathologische, klinische und genealogische Untersuchungen*. Leipzig: Thieme. [E]

Kovacs, M., Rush, A. J., Beck, A. T. and Hollon, S. D. (1981) Depressed outpatients treated with cognitive therapy or pharmacotherapy. A one year follow-up. *Arch. Gen. Psychiat.*, **38**, 33–39. [C12]

Kraepelin, E. *Psychiatrie*. Leipzig: Barth, 1896 (5. Aufl.) 1899 (6. Aufl.), 1904 (7.

Aufl.), 1909–1915 (8. Aufl.) English Edition: Dementia Praecox and Para-phrenia. Translated by Barclay, R. M. from 8th edition of Psychiatrie. Edinburgh: Livingstone, 1919. Manic depressive insanity and paranoia. In idem 8th edn, Engl. transl. Edinburgh: Livingstone, 1921. [B1, B2, B17, D3, E, E1, E3, E4, E7]

Kraepelin, E. (1913) *Psychiatrie*. III Band. *Klinsche Psychiatarie II. Teil*. Leipzig: Barth. [A, B1, B7, B9, C1, C2, C10]

Kretschmer, E. (1950) *Der sensitive Beziehungswahn*. (3. Aufl.) Berlin: Springer. [A, E, E2]

Labhardt, F. (1963) *Die schizophrenieähnlichen Emotionspsychosen. Ein Beitrag zur Abgrenzung schizophrenieartiger Zustandsbilder*. Berlin, Göttingen, Heidel-berg: Springer. [D]

Landmark, I. (1982) A manual for the Assessment of Schizophrenia. *Acta Psychiat Scand*, **65** Suppl. 298. [B1, B2, B4, B7]

Langfeldt, G. (1937) *The prognosis in schizophrenia and the factors influencing the course of the disease*. Copenhagen: Munksgaard; London: Oxford Univ. Press. [A, B4, E, E2]

Langfeldt, G. (1939) *The schizophreniform states*. Copenhagen: Munksgaard; London: Oxford Univ. Press. [A, B4, D, E, E2]

Langfeldt, G. (1956) *The prognosis in schizophrenia*. Copenhagen: Munksgaard. [A, B4, B17, E2]

Langfeldt, G. (1960) Diagnosis and prognosis of schizophrenia. *Proc. Royal Soc. Med.*, **53**, 1047–52. [B4, E2]

Langfeldt, G. (1969) Schizophrenia: diagnosis and prognosis. *Behav. Science*, **14**, 173–82. [B4]

Lenz, G. (1987) *Schizoaffektive Psychosen*. Vienna: Facultas. [D3, D4, D5, D7]

Lenz, G., Katschnig, H. and David, H. P. (1986) Symptoms, diagnosis and time in hospital: a polydiagnostic study on schizophrenia. *Psychopathology*, **19**, 253–7. [A]

Leonhard, K. (1957) *Aufteilung der endogenen Psychosen*. Akademie Verlag: Berlin. [A]

Leonhard, K. (1968) Über monopolare und bipolare endogene Psychosen. *Nervenarzt*, **39**, 104–6. [C2, C5]

Leonhard, K. (1979) *Aufteilung der endogenen Psychosen*. Berlin (DDR): Akade-mie Verlag, 1. Aufl. 1957, 5. Aufl. 1980. Engl. edition, New York: Irvington Publishers. [C2, D, D2]

Maas, J. W., Koslow, S. H., Davis, J. M., Katz, M. M., Mendels, J., Robins, E., Stokes, P. E. and Bowden, C. L. (1980) Biological component of the NIMH clinical research branch collaborative program on the psychobiology of depression: I. Background and theoretical considerations. *Psychol. Med.*, **10**, 759–76. [B8, C6, D5]

Magnan, V. (1893) Leçons cliniques. 2. édition. Bataille éd. Paris. [A, E4]

Maier, W., Philipp, M., Buller, R. and Schlegel, S. (1987) Reliability and validity of the Newcastle scales in relation to ICD–9-classification. *Acta Psychiat. Scand.*, **76**, 619–27. [C12]

Marneros, A., Deister, A. and Rhode, A. (1981) Quality of affective sympto-matology and its importance for the definition of schizoaffective disorder. *Psychopathology*, **22**, 152–60. [D3]

Marneros, A., Rhode, A., Deister, A. and Jünemann, H. (1988) Syndrome shift in long-term course of schizoaffective disorders. *Euro. Arch. Psychiat. Neurol. Sci.*, **238**, 97–104. [D3, D4]

Marneros, A., Rhode, A., Deister, A. and Risse, A. (1986) Schizoaffective disorders: The prognostic value of the affective component. In Marneros, A. and Tsuang, M. T. (eds.) *Schizoaffective psychoses*, Berlin, Heidelberg, New York: Springer. [D3]

Mattes, J. A. and Nayak, D. (1984) Lithium versus fluphenazine for prophylaxis in mainly schizophrenic schizo-affectives. *Biol. Psychiat.*, **19**, 3, 445–9. [D5]

Mayer, W. (1921) Über paraphrene Psychosen. *Z. Ges. Neurol. Psychiat.*, **71**, 187–206. [E]

McCabe, M. S. and Strömgren, E. (1975) Reactive psychoses: a family study. *Arch. Gen. Psychiat.*, **32**, 447–54. [D]

Mellor, C. S. (1982) The present status of first rank symptoms. *Brit. J. Psychiat.*, **140**, 423. [A]

Mentzos, S. (1967) *Mischzustände und mischbildhafte phasische Psychosen.* Stuttgart: Enke. [A, B14, C10]

Milln, P., Bishop, M. and Coppen, A. (1981) Urinary free cortisol and clinical classification of depressive illness. *Psychol. Med.*, **11**, 643–5. [C12]

Mirkin, A. M. and Coppen, A. (1980) Electrodermal activity in depression: clinical and biochemical correlates. *Brit. J. Psychiat.*, **137**, 93–7. [C12]

Moebius, P. J. (1893) *Abriss der Lehre von den Nervenkrankheiten.* Leipzig: A. Abel. [A]

Morel, B. A. (1860) *Traité des maladies mentales.* Paris: Masson. [B1]

Müller, C. (1981) *Psychische Erkrankungen und ihr Verlauf sowie ihre Beeinflussung durch das Alter.* Bern, Stuttgart, Wien: Hans Huber. [B14]

Nadzharow, R. A. (1967) *The clinical aspect of biological investigation of the pathogenesis of schizophrenia.* Biological research in schizophrenia, transactions of the symposium. Moscow. [B17]

Nadzharow, R. A. (1977) Verlaufsformen. In Snezhnewski, A. W. (ed.): *Schizophrenie. Multidisziplinäre Untersuchungen.* AMW der USSR. Leipzig: VEB Georg Thieme. Russ. Orig. Ausg., 1972. [B17]

Naylor, G. J., McNamee, H. B. and Moody, J. P. (1971) Changes in erythrocyte sodium and potassium on recovery from a depressive illness. *Brit. J. Psychiat.*, **118**, 219–23. [C12]

Noble, P. and Lader, M. (1972) A physiological comparison of 'endogenous' and 'reactive' depression. *Brit. J. Psychiat.*, **120**, 393–404. [C12]

Noreik, K. (1970) *Follow-up and classification of functional psychoses with special reference to reactive psychoses.* Oslo: Universitetsforlaget. [E2]

Noreik, K., Astrup, C., Dalgard, O. S. and Holmboe, R. (1967) A prolonged follow-up of acute schizophrenic and schizophreniform psychoses. *Acta Psychiat. Scand.*, **43**, 432–43 (1967). [E2]

Nunn, C. M. H. (1979) Mixed affective states and natural history of manic-depressive psychosis. *Brit. J. Psychiat.*, **134**, 153–60. [A]

Nutzinger, D. O. (1991) The concept of endogenous anxiety in the Vienna research criteria: the axial syndrome of endogenomorphic anxiety. *Psychopathology*, (in press). [C10]

Othmer, E., Penick, E. C. and Powell, B. J. (1981) *Psychiatric diagnostic interview (PDI)*. Los Angeles: Western Psychological Services. [B7]

Overall, J. E. and Hollister, L. E. (1979) Comparative evaluation of research diagnostic criteria for schizophrenia. *Arch. Gen. Psychiat.*, **36**, 1198–205. [A, B7]

Papousek, M. (1975) Chronobiologische Aspekte der Zyklothymie. *Fortschr. Neurol. Psychiat.*, **43**, 381–440. [C9, C10]

Pauleikoff, B. (1957) Atypische Psychosen. *Bibl. Psychiat.*, **99**, 51–144. [D]

Perris, C. (1966) A study of bipolar (manic-depressive) and unipolar recurrent depressive psychoses. *Acta Psychiat. Scand.*, (Suppl. 194), **42**, 1–188. [A, C5]

Perris, C. (1974) A study of cycloid psychoses. *Acta Psychiat. Scand.*, (suppl. 253). [D, D2]

Perris, C. and Brockington, I. F. (1981) Cycloid psychoses and their relation to the major psychoses. In Perris, C., Struwe, G. and Jansson, B. (eds.) *Biological Psychiatry*, pp. 447–50. Elsevier: Amsterdam. [D, D2, D5]

Philipp, M. and Maier, W. (1987) *Diagnosesysteme endogener Depressionen*. Berlin, Heidelberg, New York: Springer. [C12]

Pope, H. G. and Lipinski, J. F. (1978). Diagnosis in schizophrenia and manic-depressive illness. A reassessment of the specificity of 'schizophrenic' symptoms in the light of current research. *Arch. Gen. Psychiat.*, **35**, 811–28. [A]

Pope, H. G., Lipinski, J. F., Cohen, B. M. and Axelrod, D. T. (1980) 'Schizoaffective disorder': An invalid diagnosis? A comparison of schizoaffective disorder, schizophrenia and affective disorder. *Am. J. Psychiat.*, **137**, 921–7. [A]

Praag, W. M., van (1982) A transatlantic view of the diagnosis of depressions according to the DSM–III: I. Controversies and misunderstandings in depression diagnosis. *Compr. Psychiat.*, **23**, 315–29. [C5, C6]

Prusoff, B. A., Weissmann, M. M., Klerman, G. L. and Rounsaville, B. J. (1980) Research diagnostic criteria subtypes of depression. *Arch. Gen. Psychiat.*, **37**, 796–801. [A. C6]

Pull, C. B. and Pull, M. C. (1981) Des critères cliniques pour le diagnostic de schizophrénie. In Pichot, P. (ed.) *Actualités de la schizophrénie*. Paris: PUF. [A, B16]

Pull, C. B., Pull, M. C. and Pichot, P. (1981) L.I.C.E.T.–S: Une liste intégrée de critères d'evaluation taxinomiques pour les psychoses non-affectives. *J. de Psychiatrie Biologique et Thérapeutique*, **1**, 33, 27. [A, B16]

Pull, C. B., Pull, M. C. and Pichot, P. (1984) *L.I.C.E.T.-D 100: une liste intégrée de critères d'évaluation taxinomiques pour les dépressions. Manuel d'utilisation.* Clinique des Maladies Mentales et de l'Encéphale et Centre Hospitalier de Luxembourg. [C13]

Pull, C. B., Pull, M. C. and Pichot, P. (1987a) Des critères empiriques français pour les psychoses II. Consensus des psychiatres français et définitions provisoires. *L'Encéphale*, **XIII**, 53–7. [A, B16, E]

Pull, C. B., Pull, M. C. and Pichot, P. (1987b) Des critères empiriques français pour les psychoses. III. Algorithmes et arbre de décision. *L'Encéphale*, **XIII**, 59–66. [A, B14, B16, E, E1]

Pull, C. B., Pull, M. C. and Pichot, P. (1988) French diagnostic criteria for depression. *Psychiat. and Psychobiol.*, **3**, 321–8. [A, C13]

Rao, V. A. R. and Coppen, A. (1979) Classification of depression and response to amitriptyline treatment. *Psychol. Med.*, **9**, 321–5. [C12]

Rasch, E. (1960) *Probabilistic models for some intelligence and attainment tests.* Copenhagen: The Danish Institute for Educational Research. [C12]

Retterstøl, N. (1966) *Paranoid and paranoiac psychoses.* Oslo: Universitetsforlaget. [E2]

Retterstøl, N. (1970) *Prognosis in paranoid psychoses.* Oslo: Universitetsforlaget. [E2]

Retterstøl, N. (1975) Nosologische Aspekte der paranoiden Psychosen. *Psychiat. Clin.*, **8**, 20–30. [E2, E4]

Retterstøl, N. (1978) The Scandinavian concept of reactive psychosis, schizophreniform psychosis and schizophrenia. *Psychiat. Clin.*, **11**, 180–7. [D]

Robins, E. and Guze, S. (1970) Establishment of diagnostic validity in psychiatric illness: Its application to schizophrenia. *Am. J. Psychiat.*, **127**, 7, 983–7. [B7]

Robins, E., Munoz, R. A., Martin, S. and Gentry, K. A. (1972) Primary and secondary affective disorders. In Zubin, J. and Feyhan, F. (eds.) *Disorders of mood.* Baltimore, London: J. Hopkins Press. [A, C5]

Roth, M. (1981) Problems in the classification of affective disorder. *Acta. Psychiat. Scand.*, (Suppl. 290), **63**, 42–51. [B11, C5]

Roth, M., Gurney, C., Garside, R. F. and Kerr, T. A. (1972) Studies in the classification of affective disorders. The relationship between anxiety states and depressive illness – I. *Brit. J. Psychiat.*, **121**, 147–61. [C12]

Roth, M., Gurney, C. and Mountjoy, C. Q. (1983) The Newcastle rating scales. *Acta Psychiat. Scand.*, suppl. **310**, 42–54. [C12]

Sandifer, M. G., Wilson, I. C. and Green, L. (1966) The two-type thesis of depressive disorders. *Am. J. Psychiat.*, **123**, 93–7. [A, C10, C12]

Sartorius, N., Jablensky, A., Cooper, J. E. and Burke, J. D. (eds.) (1988) Psychiatric classification in an international perspective, with special reference to Chapt V (F) of the 10th Revision of the ICD. *Brit. J. Psychiat.*, **152**, Suppl. 1. [B6]

Schanda, H. (1987) *Paranoide Psychosen. Diagnose, Verlauf, Familienbild.* Stuttgart: Enke. [E7]

Schanda, H., Lieber, A., Küfferle, B., Gabriel, E. and Berner, P. (1986) Delusional psychosis: genetic findings as a critical variable for the validation of diagnostic criteria. *Psychopathology*, **19**, 259–66. [A]

Schanda, H., Thau, K., Küfferle, B., Kieffer, W. and Berner, P. (1984) Heterogeneity of delusional syndromes: diagnostic criteria and course prognosis. *Psychopathology*, **17**, 280–9. [E10]

Schapira, K., Roth, M., Kerr, T. A. and Gurney, C. (1972) The prognosis of affective disorders: the differentiation of anxiety states from depressive illness. *Brit. J. Psychiat.*, **121**, 175–81. [C12]

Scharfetter, C. (1975) The historical development of the concept of schizophrenia. In Lader, M. H. (ed.) Studies of schizophrenia. *Brit. J. Psychiat.*, Special Publication **10**. [B1]

Scharfetter, C., Moerbt, H. and Wing, J. K. (1976) Diagnosis of functional psychoses: comparison of clinical and computerized classifications. *Arch. Psychiat. Nervenkr.*, **222**, 61–7. [B13, C9]

Schneider, C. (1930) *Die Psychologie der Schizophrenie.* Leipzig: Thieme. [B15]

Schneider, K. (1939) *Psychischer Befund und psychiatrische Diagnose.* I. Auflage. Leipzig: G. Thieme. [A]

Schneider, K. (1950) Letter from Germany: systematic psychiatry. *Am. J. Psychiat.*, **107**, 334. [B3]

Schneider, K. (1959) *Klinische Psychopathologie.* 12., gegenüber der 8. unveränderte Aufl. Stuttgart: Thieme, 1980. Engl Edition: *Clinical Psychopathology*, translated from 3rd edn. by Hamilton, M. W. and Anderson, E. W. New York: Grune and Stratton. [B3, B8, B9, B15, C11]

Schulz, B. (1932) Zur Erbpathologie der Schizophrenie. *Z. Ges Neurol. Psychiat.*, **143**, 175–93. [E9]

Sharikov, N. M. (1977) Die Formen der Remission bei der Schizophrenie. Gerichtsmedizinische Probleme. In Snezhnewski, A. W. (ed.) *Multidisziplinäre Untersuchungen.* AMW der USSR. Leipzig: VEB Georg Thieme, p. 243. Russ. Orig. Aus., 1972. [B17]

Sheehan, D. V., Ballenger, J. and Jacobsen, G. (1980) Treatment of endogenous anxiety with phobic, hysterical and hypochondriacal symptoms. *Arch. Gen. Psychiat.*, **37**, 51–9. [C10]

Sheldon, W. H. (1940) *The varieties of human physique.* New York, London: Harper & Brothers. [B14, C10]

Slater, E. and Roth, M. (1969) *Clinical Psychiatry.* Eighth edition. Baltimore: Williams & Wilkins. [B15, C11]

Snezhnewski, A. W. (1966) Über den Verlauf und die nosologische Einheitlichkeit der Schizophrenie (Methode und Ergebnisse der Untersuchung) *Vestn. AMN SSR*, **3**,B. [B17]

Snezhnewski, A. W. (1977) Nosos et pathos schizophreniae. In Snezhnewski, A. W. (ed.) *Schizophrenie. Multidisziplinäre Untersuchungen.* AMW der UDSSR, Leipzig: Georg Thieme (Russ. Original ausg, 1972). [B17]

Specht, W. (1901) *Über den pathologischen Affect in der chronischen Paranoia. Festschrift der Erlanger Universität.* Leipzig: Böhme. [C10, E]

Spitzer, R. L., Endicott, J. and Robins, E. (1978a) Research Diagnostic Criteria: Rationale and reliability. *Arch. Gen. Psychiat.*, **35**, 773–82. [B8, C, C6, D5]

Spitzer, R. L., Endicott, J. and Robins, E. (1978b) *Research diagnostic criteria (RDC) for a selected group of functional disorders*, third edition. New York State Psychiatric Institute. [B8, C, C5, C6, D, D5,]

Spitzer, R. L., Williams, J. B. W. and Skodol, A. E. (1980) DSM–III: The major achievements and an overivew. *Am. J. Psychiat.*, **137**, 151–64. [B9, C7]

Stallone, F., Huba, G. J., Lawlor, W. G. and Fieve, H. R. (1973) Longitudinal studies of diurnal variations in depression. A sample of 643 patient days. *Brit. J. Psychiat.*, **123**, 311–8. [C10]

Stephens, J. H., Astrup, C., Carpenter, W. T. jr, Shaffer, J. W. and Goldberg, J. (1982) A comparison of nine systems to diagnose schizophrenia. *Psychiatry Research*, **6**, 127–43. [A, B7, E10]

Stephens, J. H., Astrup, C. and Mangrum, J. C. (1966) Prognostic factors in recovered and deteriorated schizophrenics. *Am. J. Psychiat.*, **122**, 1116–21. [D]

Stephens, J. H., Ota, K. Y., Carpenter, W. T. jr and Shaffer, J. W. (1980) Diagnostic criteria for schizophrenia: Prognostic implications and diagnostic overlap. *Psychiatry Research*, **2**, 1–12. [B7, E10]

Strauss, J. S. and Carpenter, W. T. jr (1974) The prediction of outcome in schizophrenia. *Arch. Gen. Psychiat.*, **31**, 37–42. [B7]

Strauss, J. S. and Carpenter, W. T. jr (1977) The prediction of outcome in schizophrenia. *Arch. Gen. Psychiat.*, **34**, 159–63. [E10]

Strauss, J. S. and Gift, T. E. (1977) Choosing an approach for diagnosing schizophrenia. *Arch. Gen. Psychiat.*, **34**, 1248–53. [B11, B12]

Taylor, M. A. (1981) *The neuropsychiatric mental status examination*. Jamaica, NY: Spectrum Publications, Inc. [B15]

Taylor, M. A. and Abrams, R. (1975a) Manic-depressive illness and good prognosis schizophrenia. *Am. J. Psychiat.*, **132**:7, 741–2. [B15]

Taylor, M. A. and Abrams, R. (1975b) A critique of the St Louis psychiatric research criteria for schizophrenia. *Am. J. Psychiat.*, **132**: 12, 1276–80. [B15, C11]

Taylor, M. A. and Abrams, R. (1978) The prevalence of schizophrenia: A reassessment using modern diagnostic criteria. *Am. J. Psychiat.*, **135**: 8, 945–8. [B14, B15, C11]

Taylor, M. A., Abrams, R. and Gaztanaga, P. (1975) Manic-depressive illness and schizophrenia: A partial validation of research diagnostic criteria utilizing neuropsychological testing. *Comp. Psychiat.*, **16**, 91–6. [B15]

Taylor, M. A., Gaztanaga, P. and Abrams, R. (1974) Manic-depressive illness and acute schizophrenia: A clinical, family history and treatment–response study. *Am. J. Psychiat.* **131**:6, 678–82. [B15, C11]

Taylor, M. A., Redfield, J. and Abrams, R. (1981) Neuropsychological dysfunction in schizophrenia and affective disease. *Biol. Psychiat.*, **16**:5, 467–78. [B15, C, C11]

Thase, M. E., Hersen, M., Bellack, A. S., Himmelhoch, J. M. and Kupfer, D. J. (1983) Validation of a Hamilton subscale for endogenomorphic depression. J. Aff. Disord., **5**, 267–278. [C12]

Thorell, L. H., Kjellman, B. F. and d'Elia, G. (1987) Electrodermal activity in relation to diagnostic subgroups and symptoms of depressive patients. *Acta Psychiat. Scand.*, **76**, 693–701. [C12]

Tölle, R. (1980) Ursachen der Melancholien und Manien. In *Die Psychologie des 20. Jahrhunderts. X.* Zürich: Kindler, pp. 484–99. [C10]

Tsuang, M. T. and Winokur, G. (1974) Criteria for subtyping schizophrenia: clinical differentiation of hebephrenic and paranoid schizophrenia. *Arch. Gen. Psychiat.*, **31**, 43–7. [E9]

Tsuang, M. T., Woolson, R. F. and Simpson, J. C. (1981) An evaluation of the Feighner criteria for schizophrenia and affective disorders using long-term, outcome data. *Psychol. Med.*, **11**, 281–7. [B7]

Vaillant, G. (1965) An historical review of the remitting schizophrenias. *J. Nerv. Ment. Dis.*, **138**, 48–56. [D]

Vlissides, D. N. and Jenner, F. A. (1982) The response of endogenously and reactively depressed patients to electroconvulsive therapy. *Brit. J. Psychiat.*, **141**, 239–42. [C12]

Waldmann, H. (1972) Die Tagesschwankungen in der Depression als rhythmisches Phänomen. *Fortschr. Neurol. Psychiat.*, **40**, 83–104. [C10]

Welner, A., Croughan, J. L. and Robins, E. (1974) The group of schizoaffective and related psychoses. Critique, record, follow-up and family studies. A persistent enigma. *Arch. Gen. Psychiat.*, **31**, 628–31. [D]

Wernicke, C. (1894) *Grundriß der Psychiatrie in klinischen Vorlesungen*. Leipzig: Thieme. [D2]

Williams, J. B. and Spitzer, R. L. (1982) Research diagnostic criteria and DSM–III. An annotated comparison. *Arch. Gen. Psychiat.*, **39**, 1283–9. [C6]

Wilmanns, K., (1932) Schizophrenie. In Bumke, O. (ed.) *Handbuch der Geisteskrankheiten 9. Band.* Berlin: Springer. Reprint, (1977). [B3]

Wimmer, A. (1916) *Psykogene sindssygdomsformer.* St. Hans Hospitals Jubilaeumsskrift. Köbenhavn. [A, E, E2]

Wing, J. K. (1980) Methodological issues in psychiatric case-identification. *Psychol. Med.*, **10**, 5–10. [B13, C9]

Wing, J. K. (1983) Use and misuse of the PSE. *Brit. J. Psychiat.*, **143**, 111–7. [B13, C9]

Wing, J. K., Babor, T., Brugha, T., Burke, J., Cooper, J. E., Giel, R., Jablenski, A., Regier, D. and Sartorius, N. (1990) SCAN. *Arch. Gen. Psychiat.*, **47**, 589–93. [B13, C9]

Wing, J. K. and Bebbington, P. (1982) Epidemiology of depressive disorders in the community. *J. Aff. Dis.*, **4**, 331–45. [A, C9]

Wing, J. K., Birley, J. L. T., Cooper, J. C., Graham, P. and Isaacs, A. D. (1967) Reliability of a procedure for measuring and classifying 'present psychiatric state'. *Brit. J. Psychiat.*, **1**, 499. [B13, C9]

Wing, J. K., Cooper, J. E. and Sartorius, N. (1974) *Measurement and classification of psychiatric symptoms.* Cambridge: Cambridge University Press. [A, B13, C, C9, E8]

Wing, J. K., Mann, S. A., Leff, J. P. and Nixon, J. M. (1978) The concept of a 'case' in psychiatric population surveys. *Psychol. Med.*, **8**, 203–17. [B13, C9]

Wing, J. K., Nixon, J., von Cranach, M. and Strauss, A. (1977) Further developments of the PSE and CATEGO system. *Arch. Psychiat. Nervenkr.*, **224**, 151–60. [B13, C9]

Wing, J. K., and Sturt, E. (1978) *The PSE-ID-CATEGO system, supplementary manual.* London: Med. Research Council. [B13, C9]

Winokur, G. (1977) Delusional disorder (paranoia). *Compr. Psychiat.*, **18**, 511–21. [E, E6, E9, E10]

Winokur, G. (1981) Classification: The bridge of the River Styx. *Adv. Biol. Psychiat.*, **7**, 14–25. Basel: Karger. [C5]

Winokur, G. (1982) The development and validity of familial subtypes in primary unipolar depression. *Pharmacopsychiatry*, **15**, 142–6. [C5]

Winokur, G., Clayton, P. J. and Reich, T. (1969) *Manic depressive illness.* St. Louis: C. V. Mosby Company. [C5]

World Health Organization (WHO) (1973) *The International Pilot Study of Schizophrenia (IPSS).* Geneva: WHO. [B3, B13, C9, E8]

World Health Organization (WHO) (1979) *Schizophrenia: An international follow-up study.* New York: J. Wiley & Sons. [E10]

Young, M. A., Scheftner, W. A., Klerman, G. L., Andreasen, N. C. and Hirschfeld, R. M. A. (1986) The endogenous subtype of depression: a study of its internal construct validity. *Brit. J. Psychiat.*, **148**, 257–67. [C12]

Young, M. A., Tanner, M. A. and Meltzer, H. Y. (1982) Operational definition of schizophrenia. What do they identify? *J. Nervous and Mental Disease*, **170**, 443–7. [A]

Zimmermann, M., Coryell, W., Pfohl, B. and Stangl, D. (1987) An American validation study of the Newcastle diagnostic scale. II. Relationship with clinical, demographic, familial and psychosocial features. *Brit. J. Psychiat.*, **150**, 526–32. [C12]

Zimmermann, M., Pfohl, B., Stangl, D. and Coryell, W. (1986) An American validation study of the Newcastle diagnostic scale. I. Relationship with the dexamethasone suppression test. *Brit. J. Psychiat.*, **149**, 627–30. [C12]

Zisook, S., Glick, M. jr, Jaffe, K. and Overall, J. E. (1980) Research criteria for the diagnosis of depression. *Psychiatry Research*, **2**, 13–23. [C6]